The Complete Keto Diet Cookbook For Beginners 2019

Quick and Simple Ketogenic Recipes For Smart People | Lose Weight And Become Healthy With The Keto Diet

Table of Content

INTRODUCTION 6
The Ketogenic Diet, What Is It? 6
The Benefits of the Keto Diet 7
Here's What You Can and Can't Eat on the Keto Diet 9
Keto Macros 14
INTRO TO RECIPES 15
Snacks and Appetizers 15
    Zucchini Parmesan Chips 15
    Cinnamon Granola 16
    Italian AntiPasto Skewers 17
    Tzatziki Avocado Salmon Rolls 18
    Taco Cups 19
    Vietnamese Chicken Meatball with Dipping Sauce 20
    Bacon Wrapped Jalapeno Poppers 21
    Chicken Satay Skewers with Peanut Sauce 22
    Cajun Shrimp with Cucumbers and Avocado 24
    Brie Bites with Raspberry Topping 25
    Spinach Artichoke Dip Pull-Apart Rolls 27
    Cauliflower Hummus 29
    Fudgy Brownie 30
Smoothies 31
    Micro-nutrient Greens Matcha Smoothie 31
    Mocha Smoothie 32
    Raspberry Coconut Smoothie 33
    Frosted Vanilla Blackberry Lemonade Smoothie 34
    Chocolate Berry Smoothie 35
    Strawberry Black Currant Smoothie 36
    Minty Green Protein Smoothie Shake 37
    Turmeric "Golden" Milkshake Turmeric 38
    Chocolate Coconut Smoothie 39
Breakfast 40
    Brie and Berries Crepe Breakfast 40
    California Chicken Omelet 41
    Cream Cheese Pancakes 42
    Mexican Frittata 43
    Raspberry & Cream Crepes 44
    Cauliflower Hash Browns 45

- Shakshuka – Eggs Poached in Tomato Sauce 46
- Chia Berry Yogurt Parfaits 47
- Filipino Breakfast Torta Omelet 48
- Breakfast "Crunch" Cereal 49
- Greek Spinach, Herb and Feta Wrap 50
- Smoked Salmon Breakfast Salad 51
- Breakfast Sausage with Guacamole Stacks 52
- Egg Crust Breakfast Pizza 53
- Cheesy Italian Omelet 54

Lunch 55
- Asian Cashew Chicken Lettuce Wraps 55
- Zucchini Crust Grilled Cheese 56
- Poke with Ahi Tuna and Citrus 57
- Chicken Quesadilla 58
- Mongolian Beef Bowl 59
- Quick Spicy Tuna Rolls 60
- Buddha Bowl 61
- Fish Tacos 62
- Creamy Butternut Squash Soup 64
- Cobb Salad 65
- Philly Cheesesteak Stuffed Peppers 66
- Sri Lankan Spicy Chili Cabbage Stir Fry 67
- Chicken Enchilada Bowl 68
- Zucchini Noodles with Garlic Shrimp 69
- Salmon Stuffed Avocado 70
- Chipotle Steak Bowl 71
- Grilled Lemon Herb Mediterranean Chicken Salad 72
- Blackened Steak Salad 74
- Tuna Cakes 76
- Hearty Chicken Soup 77
- Egg Roll in a Bowl 78

Dinner 79
- General Tso's Chicken 79
- Philly Cheesesteak Stuffed Peppers 81
- Cauliflower Rice with King Crab 82
- Chicken Tetrazzini 83
- Salmon Patties 85
- Jamaican Curry Chicken 86
- Creamy Asparagus and Shrimp Alfredo 87

Shredded Chicken Chili 88
Garlic Butter Brazilian Steak 89
Pork Chops Smothered in Caramelized Onion & Bacon 90
Creamy Garlic Chicken Soup 91
Roasted Lemon Chicken 92
Cheesy Zucchini Gratin Casserole 93
Classic Italian Meatballs 94
Italian Sausage with Peppers and Onions in Marinara Sauce 95
Easy Shrimp Scampi 96
Beef Stuffed Zucchini Boats 97
Rainbow Vegetable Noodles 98
Zucchini Noodles with Garlic Shrimp 99
Maple Walnut Crusted Salmon 100
Conclusion & FAQ 101

Introduction

Welcome to the world of keto! I know that as a beginner just starting out on the ketogenic diet, it can be so exciting, interesting but also overwhelming. That feeling of being overwhelming is probably due to all the very specific guidelines you HAVE to follow to successfully get into ketosis. But there's no need to worry! Now that you have my cookbook, I'll help you transition from your current diet smoothly into ketosis so you can get the results you want.

My cookbook will provide you with all the basic info you need in order to understand the keto diet, including the science behind ketosis, what you can and can't eat on this diet, along with practical tips. And of course, my cookbook wouldn't be complete without my delicious Keto-friendly recipes that are perfect for beginners like you!

Now, let's get into what makes the Keto Diet so different from the rest.

The Ketogenic Diet, What Is It?

Simply put, the ketogenic diet is a low-carb diet that is high in fat and includes a moderate amount of protein. After you follow the diet for a while, your body will go into a metabolic state which is known as ketosis. While in ketosis, your liver will switch from is regular function and start to produce ketones. These ketones will move glucose out of the way and become your body's main source of energy.

So why is everyone going crazy about the diet? Well, for starters it will change how your body functions in the most natural way and change the way you view food as fuel.

And this is important since the keto diet is based on the premise that your body lags as a sugar burner and works better as a fat burner.

The Transition: From Sugar to Fat
Your body automatically produces glucose and insulin soon after you enjoy a yummy, yet carb pack treats like a sweet piece of cake or buttered bagel. Why does your body choose to produce glucose? It just so happens to be the easiest molecule for your body to convert and use as energy. It's also the main reason why your body prefers this energy source because it's so quick and easy. Now, your body produces insulin to process the glucose in your bloodstream as it goes through your body.

This sounds really efficient, right? It's fast and your body can get the energy it needs quickly so you can function. But the problem with this easy process is that your body can only use a limited amount of glucose as its main energy source. Anything else will be converted into fat and stored. And when your glucose levels start running low again, your body will also tell your brain you need to hurry up and grab a sugary or carb-filled snack to refill that energy source.

Now you see, this dangerous cycle of consuming unhealthy foods for energy can lead to excess body fat and of course health problems. The best way to stop this terrible cycle is to turn your body into a fat burner! And you can do this on the keto diet.

Once you lower your carb intake enough, your body will start to look for a different energy source – and this means ketosis is about to begin! When your body is in ketosis, it will produce ketones that only occur when the liver breaks down excess fat cells.

You're probably thinking why doesn't my body naturally do this if it's healthier for me? Well, when your body produces insulin, ketosis is essentially blocked because insulin prevents any fat cells from entering your bloodstream and from there they're just stored in your body.

But when you lower your carb intake, your glucose and blood sugar levels dramatically drop and in turn eventually lower your insulin levels. This opens a way for fat cells to finally release the water they're storing (aka water weight) and enter your bloodstream heading straight to your liver.

Turning your useless fat cells into your go-to energy source is the main goal of the keto diet. Just remember, you won't get into ketosis by starving your body of food. You can only enter a state of ketosis by laying off the carbohydrates and sugar.

And don't worry, you won't miss those two when you start noticing all the physical and mental changes, which I'll get into next!

The Benefits of the Keto Diet

You can change your whole life with the right diet and the keto diet is no exception! I'm sure you've read plenty of success stories online or even personally heard about how great this diet is from someone close. The keto diet isn't a fad, it's a new kind of lifestyle that provides real results and benefits – including the following;

Shed the Pounds
The most popular reasons why people look to the keto diet is to lose weight. It happens to be one of the most effective ways to shed the pounds since the diet will force your body to use excess fat as an energy source. Helping you burn unwanted fat, reach your weight loss goals and most importantly turn your body into a fat burning machine!

Control Over Your Blood Sugar Levels
A lot of people have to deal with diabetes every day of their lives due to their body's inability to handle insulin. If you happen to be one of them, the keto diet can help. It will

naturally lower your blood sugar levels because you'll be cutting carbs and producing less glucose.

The keto diet is also a huge benefit to those of you who are pre-diabetic or have Type II diabetes. It will help you maintain healthier blood sugar levels and have more control over your life.

As with any dietary changes when you have diabetes, you'll need to discuss it with your doctor before you make choosing the keto diet.

Lower Insulin Resistance
People suffer from Type II diabetes due to insulin resistance. The ketogenic diet can help individuals lower their insulin levels down to a healthier range and get out of the high-risk group going to develop diabetes.

Clarity and Better Focus
Ever have a mental fog that lasts all day? That lack of clarity and focus was probably a side effect of eating too many carbs. Once you start the ketogenic diet, you'll finally experience a clear increase in your mental performance. In fact, plenty of people are switching to keto to better their daily focus and clear their thinking.

And to think, this is all because ketones are a wonderful source of fuel for your brain!

Boost in Energy
You already know that the keto diet will turn your body fat into an energy source, but did you know it will also increase your energy levels?

When you're just consuming carbs for energy, you will cause your blood sugar levels to rise and fall, and then feel the crash later. The keto diet will give you a much more reliable energy source and keep you more energized all day long!

Control Over Your Appetite
On your last diet, you probably noticed yourself reaching for snacks throughout the day. This was mainly because you were eating so many empty carbs, but on the keto diet, you'll stay fuller longer. It's mainly because fats ward off the hunger pains and they'll leave your body in a more satiated state.

In the end, the keto diet will help lessen the craving for sugary and carb-filled foods and you can avoid feeling weak from not constantly snacking.

Lower Cholesterol & Blood Pressure
The ketogenic diet also helps to improve the levels of triglyceride and cholesterol in your body. Research has shown that a diet that is high in fat and low in carbs will give you an increase in HDL (which is the good cholesterol) and decrease the LDL (the bad kind of

cholesterol). Other studies have also shown that low-carb diets improve blood pressure much better than other traditional diets.

Treatment for Epilepsy

Since the early 1900s, the ketogenic diet has been used to treat people with epilepsy. Even today, it's used as a way to treat children who suffer from uncontrolled epilepsy.

And for those who are adults with epilepsy, the keto diet will give you a chance to take fewer medications, which is a huge plus.

Here's What You Can and Can't Eat on the Keto Diet

As with any diet out there, you have to know what you can't and can eat. With that being said, the keto diet has its own set of restrictions in order to get you into ketosis. Just remember that the end goal is to turn your body into a fat burning machine. And for that to happen you need to drastically reduce your carb in sugar intake. But don't worry, once you're in ketosis you'll find yourself craving sugary foods and carbs less and looking for more healthier options.

Now let's finally see what you can't and can eat below.

What to Avoid
Grains and Carbs

Grains and carbs are exactly what you need to avoid on the keto diet, so don't add these to your shopping list:

- Wheat
- Buckwheat
- Beer
- Corn
- Pasta
- Rice
- Bread
- Barley
- Quinoa
- Cereal
- Pastries

Fruits

Most fruits are high in carbs, whether they're fresh, frozen or juiced.

- Apples
- Bananas

- Oranges
- Tangerines
- Grapes
- Pineapples
- Mangos
- Papayas
- Dates

Root Veggies and Tubers

Start avoiding these starchy root vegetables and tubers from now on:

- Potatoes
- Yams
- Sweet potatoes
- Carrots
- Parsnips
- All by-products

Sugar

Be vigilant and avoid all kinds of sugar and its by-products because they will quickly throw you out of ketosis.

- Cane sugar
- Agave syrup
- Ice creams
- Cakes
- Puddings
- Soft-drinks
- Sports drinks
- Candy
- Chocolate
- Breakfast cereal
- Juice
- Artificial Sweeteners

Low-Fat, Low-Carb Dairy Products

Dairy products that are low in fat tend to have more carbs and sugar. On the other hand, low-carb dairy products can contain artificial additives. So make sure you avoid both.

- Low-fat milk
- Low-fat yogurt
- Diet soda

Trans Fats, Refined Fats, and Oils

Toss these (if you have them) and avoid these trans fats, refined fats and oils from now on.
- Margarine
- Spreadable butter alternatives
- Cottonseed oil
- Soybean oil
- Grapeseed oil
- Corn oil
- Safflower oil
- Sunflower oil

Processed Foods
Steer clear of these products and preservatives found in processed foods.
- Carrageenan - found in almond milk-based products
- Wheat gluten
- MSG - Added to whey protein products
- Sulphites - found in dried fruits and gelatin
- BPAs – they're often not labeled

Food You Can Enjoy
The can't list above is pretty long, but there are plenty of foods you can eat on the keto diet. Below is a quick rundown of everything you can enjoy!

Seafood
Avoid farm-raised fish and choose fresh, wild-caught seafood for your meals.
- Shrimp
- Lobster
- Tuna
- Halibut
- Mahi Mahi
- Catfish
- Oysters
- Salmon
- Mackerel
- Cod
- Mussels
- Clams
- Crab
- Squid

- Octopus

Meat and Protein
Always choose organic, pasture-raised, grass-fed meats when you can.
- Beef
- Poultry
- Pork
- Lamb
- Goat
- Organs
- Bacon
- Eggs

Low-Sugar Fruits
Here are a few fruits you can have on the Keto Diet, in moderation of course.
- Strawberries
- Blueberries
- Raspberries
- Cherries
- Mulberries
- Cranberries
- Avocados
- Watermelon
- Cantaloupe
- Coconut (meat)
- Peaches
- Lemons

Low-Carb Vegetables
Rule of thumb to remember while shopping- stick to vegetables that grow above the ground. They're really low in carbs.
- Celery
- Asparagus
- Chives
- Bok choy
- Eggplant
- Lettuce
- Kale
- Brussel Sprouts
- Spinach

- Bell Peppers
- Broccoli
- Radicchio
- Zucchini
- Avocado
- Green Beans
- Cauliflower
- Cucumber
- Radishes
- Mushrooms
- Cabbage
- Endives
- Swiss chard

Fats and Oils

Concentrate on getting most of your fat from natural sources. If needed, you can also supplement it with monounsaturated fats, saturated fats, and polyunsaturated omega-3s.

- Olive Oil
- Coconut Oil
- Butter
- Ghee
- Avocado Oil
- Macadamia nuts
- Lard
- Duck fat
- Beef Oil
- Canola Oil

High-Fat Dairy

Only fill your fridge with full-fat dairy products such as the following:

- Heavy cream
- Cream cheese
- Sour cream
- Full-fat yogurt
- Mayonnaise
- Cottage cheese
- Hard cheeses like parmesan, swiss, feta, and cheddar
- Soft cheeses like brie, mozzarella, Monterey Jack, and blue cheese

Nuts

Nuts are definitely a snack you can have on this diet, just enjoy them in moderation.
- Walnuts
- Peanuts
- Pine nuts
- Almonds
- Pecans
- Brazil nuts
- Macadamia nuts
- Hazelnuts

Sweeteners

If you ever need to make a drink, dessert or snack a little sweeter, you can reach for these safe, low-glycemic sweeteners like these:
- Stevia
- Erythritol
- Sucralose
- Xylitol
- Yacon Syrup
- Monk fruit
- Any other kind of low-carb sweeteners on the market

Keto Macros

So, what are macros? There the key to being successful on the keto diet and the main source of calories in your everyday diet. In total, there are three macros that you need to watch carefully - fats, protein, and carbs.

Since the keto diet is high in fat, that's where you'll get a majority of your daily calories. To keep things in check, the general ratio of macros you need on the keto diet is 70% fat, 25% protein, and 5% carbohydrates.

When you finally kick start your keto diet, your daily intake of net carbs shouldn't exceed no more than 20g. No excuses. Even if you calculate beforehand and you're recommended daily macro carb count is 27g for example, you still need to stay at below 20g when you start out.

Intro to Recipes

Say goodbye to carbs and hello to more fulfilling meals with the recipes that I have for you below! Just look through my recipe list and get ready to make cream cheese pancakes for breakfast, a zesty roasted lemon chicken for dinner, zucchini parmesan chips and so much more!

Snacks and Appetizers

Zucchini Parmesan Chips

Such a good way to enjoy your veggies! And I'm sure the pickiest of picky eaters will enjoy this healthy snack!

Prep Time: 5 Minutes
Cook Time: 20 Minutes
Total Time: 25 Minutes
Serves: 5-6

Ingredients:
- 4 small zucchinis
- 1 to 1 ½ cups of Parmesan - romano blend cheese (or your favorite cheese)

Optional:
- Sugar free marinara sauce, for dipping

Directions:
1. Preheat the oven to 425 degrees F
2. Slice each of the zucchini into slices, about ¼ inch thick
3. Prep a large baking sheet with tin foil or parchment paper
4. Spread the sliced zucchini rounds out on to the baking sheet, season with salt and pepper - Make sure to season to taste depending on the flavor of the cheese
5. Then sprinkle the cheese evenly over each zucchini round covering each one
6. Bake for about 15 to 20 minutes or until the cheese is golden brown
7. Serve with sugar free marinara sauce
8. Serve warm and enjoy!

Recipe Note – Try mixing things up with zucchini and yellow squash. Both vegetables are amazing in this recipe.

Macros Per Serving – Calories:68 |Total Fat: 4g | Protein: 6g| **Net Carbs: 1g**

Cinnamon Granola

Enjoy it on the go, dry or like your favorite cereal!

Prep Time: 5 Minutes
Cook Time: 20 Minutes
Total Time: 25 Minutes
Serves: 4

Ingredients:
- 5 tbsp flax seed meal
- 5 tbsp unsweetened coconut flakes
- 1 tbsp chia seeds
- 1 ½ oz. nuts of your choice – we used pecans, walnuts, and almonds
- 4 tbsp sugar free maple syrup

Optional:
- 1 ½ tsp ground cinnamon

Directions:
1. Preheat oven to 350 degrees F
2. In a bowl, combine the coconut flakes, flax seed meal, chia seeds, nuts of your choice and maple syrup
3. Prepare a baking sheet and spread out the mixture to make one layer
4. Sprinkle with the cinnamon
5. Bake for 20-22 minutes
6. Allow to cool so the granola hardens
7. Enjoy!

Macros Per Serving – Calories:175 |Total Fat: 17g | Protein: 6g| **Net Carbs: 3g**

Italian AntiPasto Skewers

Oh, these antipasto skewers are so easy to make and are perfect for any dinner party!

Prep Time: 10 Minutes

Total Time: 10 Minutes

Serves: 16

Ingredients:
- 8 prosciutto slices
- 16 ciliegine (1 inch) mozzarella balls
- 16 sun dried tomatoes, in oil
- 16 fresh basil leaves

Directions:
1. Cut the prosciutto slices in half
2. Fold up the prosciutto and place one sun dried tomato, one basil leaf, and one mozzarella ball on top of it
3. Skewer each one onto the toothpick

Macros Per Serving – Calories:60|Total Fat: 4g | Protein: 6g| **Net Carbs: 1g**

Tzatziki Avocado Salmon Rolls

Tzatziki Avocado Salmon Rolls are the perfect party appetizer. They're delicious, easy to make, and healthy. Plus, you can make them ahead of time!

Prep Time: 15 Minutes
Total Time: 15 Minutes
Serves: 4

Ingredients:
- 2 tbsp minced chives, divided plus extra whole chives for garnish
- Juice from ¼ lime
- ½ ripe avocado, peeled and sliced
- 5 oz. wild smoked salmon
- 1 English cucumber, cut into 8 thin strips, remove the seeds and 12 rounds
- 2 tbsp sesame seeds, or mix of white and black
- 2 tbsp extra thick Tzatziki sauce

Directions:
1. In a small bowl, mix together the tzatziki, 1 tsp of minced chives, and the lime juice.
2. Lay a piece of plastic wrap, about 16 inch. long down
3. Place the smoked salmon on top of the plastic, overlapping the pieces to make a 12" x 7" rectangle. Pat them all down gently so that they stick together.
4. Spread the tzatziki over the salmon, top with the cucumber strips, and sprinkle the remaining chives over the top
5. Using the plastic, roll the salmon tightly then sprinkle the sesame seeds over the top
6. Refrigerate the roll for 15 minutes to slice the rolls easier
7. Slice the salmon roll into 12 pieces, place them on cucumber slices, and top with 2 small chives each
8. Serve!

Macros Per Serving – Calories:139 |Total Fat: 8g | Protein: 9g| **Net Carbs: 3g**

Taco Cups

Who doesn't love tacos?! Make your guests happy with these bite size taco cups filled with ground beef, salsa and cheese.

Prep Time: 10 Minutes
Cook Time: 20 Minutes
Total Time: 30 Minutes
Serves: 8

Ingredients:
- 3 cloves garlic, minced
- 1 lb. ground beef
- 1 tsp chili powder
- ½ tsp ground cumin
- ½ tsp paprika
- Kosher salt
- Freshly ground black pepper

To Serve:
- Sour cream
- Chopped cilantro
- Chopped tomatoes

Directions:
1. Preheat oven to 375 degrees F
2. Line a large baking sheet with parchment paper
3. With a spoon add about a tbsp of cheese a few inches apart
4. Bake until the cheese is bubbly and edges are golden, about 6 minutes
5. Then allow to cool on baking sheet for a minute
6. In the meantime, grease bottom of muffin tin with cooking spray, then carefully pick up melted cheese slices and place on bottom of muffin tin, allow to cool for 10 minutes
7. In a large skillet over medium heat, add the olive oil
8. Once heated, add the onion and cook, stirring occasionally, until soft, about 5 minutes
9. Stir in garlic then add in the ground beef, breaking up the meat with a wooden spoon, cook until beef is no longer pink, about 6 minutes, then drain fat
10. Season with cumin, chili powder, paprika, salt, and pepper
11. Transfer the cheese cups to a serving platter and fill with cooked ground beef
12. Top with sour cream, avocado, cilantro, and tomatoes

Macros Per Serving – Calories:126|Total Fat: 6g | Protein: 15g| **Net Carbs: 1g**

Vietnamese Chicken Meatball with Dipping Sauce

These spicy and tangy Vietnamese Chicken Meatballs are the perfect appetizer and can be served up on top of a crispy bed of lettuce or alone.

Prep Time: 15 Minutes
Cook Time: 25 Minutes
Total Time: 40 Minutes
Serves: 4

Ingredients:

For the Meatballs:
- 1 (10 lbs) chicken thigh, roughly chopped
- 4 spring onions, roughly chopped
- 2 red chilis
- 1 ½ tbsp garlic paste
- 1 ½ tsp ginger paste
- ½ cup coriander leaves loosely packed
- 1 tbsp sesame oil
- 2 tbsp almond meal
- 1 ½ tsp salt

For the Sauce:
- ¼ cup fish sauce
- ¼ cup rice wine vinegar
- 1 tbsp xylitol
- 1 small red chili thinly sliced
- 2 tbsp lime juice
- 1 tsp garlic paste

Directions:
1. Preheat the oven to 365 degrees F and line a baking tray with baking paper
2. In a food processor or powerful blender, blend all meatball ingredients (chicken thigh, spring onions, red chilis, garlic paste, ginger paste, coriander, sesame oil, almond meal and salt) together until the chicken is broken down - It's ok to have slightly larger pieces of chicken
3. Roll tbsp size balls of the meatball mixture and then place the meatballs onto the baking tray about 2cm apart
4. Bake for 20-25 minutes or until cooked through - alternatively, you can fry the meatballs in a large pan with coconut oil until cooked through
5. In the meantime, prepare the dressing by whisking together the fish sauce, rice wine vinegar, xylitol, red chili, lime juice and garlic paste in a bowl
6. Serve the chicken meatballs immediately

Macros Per Serving – Calories:383|Total Fat: 26g | Protein: 23g| **Net Carbs: 6g**

Bacon Wrapped Jalapeno Poppers

It only takes 3 ingredients to make the best bacon wrapped jalapeño poppers in town!

Prep Time: 15 Minutes
Cook Time: 25 Minutes
Total Time: 40 Minutes
Serves: 20

Ingredients:
- 10 jalapeños, stems cut and sliced lengthwise, seeds removed
- 10 slices bacon
- ½ container 8 oz. cream cheese

Directions:
1. Preheat the oven to 400 degrees
2. Lay out the jalapeño, spoon about a tbsp of cream cheese in the middle of each one, set aside
3. Cut each bacon in half, wrap a half of bacon around one stuffed jalapeno then secure with a toothpick
4. Bake in the oven for 25 minutes, you can broil the last few minutes for a crispier finish
5. Plate and serve!

Macros Per Serving – Calories:67|Total Fat: 6g | Protein: 1g| **Net Carbs: 0g**

Chicken Satay Skewers with Peanut Sauce

Marinated in coconut milk and curry, this easy chicken satay recipe is served up with a delicious Thai inspired peanut sauce.

Prep Time: 15 Minutes, 6 H marinating
Cook Time: 15 Minutes
Total Time: 30 Minutes + 6 H
Serves: 4

Ingredients:
- 2 boneless skinless chicken breasts
- 10 wooden skewers
- 1 scallion thinly sliced

For the marinade:
- ½ cup full-fat coconut milk
- 3 cloves garlic minced
- ½ tsp curry powder
- ½ tsp salt
- ½ tsp ground black pepper
- ¼ tsp cayenne powder

For the peanut sauce:
- ¼ cup all-natural creamy peanut butter
- 3 cloves garlic minced
- 2 tbsp sesame oil
- 1 tbsp olive oil
- 1 tbsp soy sauce
- 1 tbsp lime juice

Directions:
1. In a large bowl, combine the coconut milk, minced garlic, curry powder, salt, pepper and cayenne pepper and stir until well-mixed
2. Slice the chicken breasts into 1 inch chunks, add them to the marinade, stirring to coat well Cover and refrigerate for at least 6 hours
3. Once the chicken is ready, thread chicken pieces onto the skewers, leaving about half of each skewer empty for handling and then place them in a single layer on a large baking sheet
4. Bake at 450 degrees F for 10 minutes, flip the skewers, and then bake for another 5 minutes or until cooked through
5. In the meantime, create the sauce by adding the creamy peanut butter, minced garlic, sesame oil, olive oil, soy sauce and lime juice to a small saucepan, whisk

together over medium-low heat until smooth, then keep warm over low heat, stirring occasionally.
6. To serve, transfer the chicken skewers onto a serving plate, brush peanut sauce over the chicken and garnish with sliced scallions and optionally black pepper
7. Serve while warm

Recipe Note: Alternatively, you can grill the chicken skewers.
Macros Per Serving – Calories:330 |Total Fat: 20g | Protein: 30g| **Net Carbs: 2g**

Cajun Shrimp with Cucumbers and Avocado

These shrimp appetizers are made with plump and juicy Cajun shrimp over creamy avocado on top of a crisp slice of cucumber! And they're a delicious mouthful!

Prep Time: 15 Minutes
Cook Time: 5 Minutes
Total Time: 20 Minutes
Serves: 22

Ingredients:

For the cajun shrimp:
- 1 lb large shrimp peeled and deveined
- 2 garlic cloves finely minced
- 1 tbsp cilantro finely chopped, plus more to garnish
- 1 tsp paprika
- ½ tsp cayenne pepper
- ½ tsp sea salt
- ¼ tsp black pepper
- 2 tbsp olive oil divided

For the avocado spread:
- 1 avocado
- ¼ tsp salt
- 1 tbsp lime juice plus more to squeeze over finished appetizers
- 1 English cucumber sliced into 22 rings

Directions:
1. Place the shrimp in a large mixing bowl and pat dry with paper towels
2. Once dry, add minced garlic, 1 tbsp cilantro, 1 tsp paprika, 1/2 tsp cayenne pepper, 1/2 tsp salt, 1/4 tsp black pepper and 1 tbsp olive oil, stir well to combine
3. Place a large heavy pan over medium/high heat, add 1 tbsp olive oil
4. Once heated, add the shrimp in a single layer and sauté 2 minutes per side or until cooked through
5. In a small bowl, mash together 1 avocado, 1/4 tsp salt and 1 tbsp lime juice until creamy, then divide the avocado mixture over 20-22 cucumber slices.
6. Squeeze fresh lime juice over each of the shrimp avocado bites and then garnish with finely chopped cilantro
7. Serve!

Recipe Notes: If you're making this recipe in advance, you can cover and refrigerate it for up to 4 hours before serving

Macros Per Serving – Calories:49 |Total Fat: 2g | Protein: 4g| **Net Carbs: 1g**

Brie Bites with Raspberry Topping

Impress your guests with a tray of these Brie Bites with Raspberry topping! Made with only 8 ingredients, they'll be ready in just 10 minutes of prep and will wow your guests.

Prep Time: 10 Minutes
Cook Time: 20 Minutes
Total Time: 30 Minutes
Serves: 36

Ingredients:
- 2 cups shredded mozzarella cheese
- 2 oz. cream cheese
- 1 cup almond flour
- ¼ cup coconut flour
- 1 egg, room temperature
- 1 tsp baking powder
- 4 oz. brie cheese
- 2 tbsp no sugar added raspberry jam
- ¼ cup frozen raspberries chopped
- Powdered sweetener like stevia, optional

Directions:
1. Preheat oven to 350 degrees F and grease the holes of the 2 mini muffin tins with the cooking spray
2. Place the cheese in a microwave-safe bowl, microwave one minute and stir, then microwave for 30 seconds, and stir - All the cheese should be melted, microwave 30 more seconds until it's uniform and it looks like fondue
3. In a food processor, add in the cheese, almond flour, egg, coconut flour, and baking powder, mix using the dough blade until the dough is a uniform color
4. Once the dough is a uniform color use a small cookie scoop to divide the dough between 36 holes of 2 mini muffin tins make
5. Use your thumbs to make an indent in the center of each - it helps to wet your thumbs with water so the dough doesn't stick
6. Bake for 20 minutes until puffed up and golden brown
7. Immediately after removing the cooked dough cups from the oven, add a cube of brie into the center of each cup
8. Then use a butter knife to pop out the appetizer bites and transfer them to a serving platter
9. Top with jam, chopped raspberries, and powdered sweetener

Recipe Notes:
You can also mix the dough in a medium bowl with a wooden spoon if you don't have a food processor, but you may need to place the dough onto wax paper and knead it by hand to thoroughly mix.

Macros Per Serving – Calories:59 |Total Fat: 4g | Protein: 3g| **Net Carbs: 1g**

Spinach Artichoke Dip Pull-Apart Rolls

Oh, you and your guests will love this recipe for pull apart rolls with a creamy spinach artichoke dip right in the center!

Prep Time: 30 Minutes
Cook Time: 20 Minutes
Total Time: 50 Minutes
Serves: 12

Ingredients:

For the rolls:
- 6 oz. cream cheese
- 2 ¼ cups shredded mozzarella cheese
- 3 large eggs
- 2 ¼ tbsp aluminum free baking powder
- 1 cup + ½ tbsp almond flour

For the dip:
- 1 (7 oz.) can artichoke hearts, drained and finely chopped
- 4 oz. cream cheese
- ½ cup mozzarella
- ¼ cup parmesan cheese
- ¼ cup sour cream
- 1 ½ cups fresh spinach, finely chopped
- 1 clove garlic, minced
- ¼ onion, minced
- ¼ tsp salt
- 1/8 tsp pepper

Directions:
1. Preheat the oven to 400 degrees F
2. In a small pot over low heat, add the cream cheese and mozzarella, and melt together – the finish product should resemble a thick gooey paste
3. Transfer the melted cheeses to a large bowl, add in the baking powder, almond flour, and eggs Mix well until smooth, then refrigerate for 10-20 minutes
4. Once cooled, roll into 12 balls and chill in the refrigerator for at least another 10 minutes until set
5. While the dough is chilling, prepare the spinach dip by adding the artichoke hearts, cream cheese, parmesan cheese, sour cream, fresh spinach, minced garlic, minced onion salt and pepper in a large bowl, mix well to combine

6. Place the dough balls around the edge of the skillet touching on each side, then fill the center with the spinach dip
7. Bake for 17-20 minutes until the rolls are fluffy, golden brown, and cooked through
8. Serve!

Macros Per Serving – Calories:239 |Total Fat: 20g | Protein: 12g| **Net Carbs: 3g**

Cauliflower Hummus

Yummy cauliflower hummus is an amazing snack and tastes very similar to ordinary hummus. Enjoy with celery or your favorite low-carb veggies.

Prep Time: 10 Minutes
Cook Time: 40 Minutes
Total Time: 50 Minutes
Serves: 4

Ingredients:

- 1 medium cauliflower
- ⅓ cup tahini
- 2 tsp cumin
- 1 tbsp olive oil
- 1 tsp salt
- ½ tsp smoked paprika
- 2 cloves garlic, crushed

Directions:

1. Preheat the oven to 355 degrees F
2. Remove all the florets from the cauliflower
3. Place the cauliflower on a baking tray, and season with cumin
4. Bake for 30 minutes
5. Remove the cauliflower, and place into a blender, blend until chunky
6. Add in the tahini, crushed garlic, paprika, and salt, blend again
7. Transfer to a small bowl
8. Covering with olive oil and coriander
9. Serve!

Macros Per Serving – Calories:183 |Total Fat: 15g | Protein: 6g| **Net Carbs: 4g**

Fudgy Brownie

These super easy to make brownies are low in carbs, creamy, and of course fudgy!

Prep Time: 10 Minutes
Cook Time: 20 Minutes
Total Time: 30 Minutes
Serves: 8

Ingredients:

- ½ cup almond flour
- 3 eggs at room temperature
- 12 tbsp butter softened
- ¼ cup dark cocoa powder
- 2 oz. dark chocolate
- ¾ cup erythritol
- ½ tsp baking powder

Directions:

1. Preheat oven to 350 degrees F
2. Line parchment paper in an 8 x 8-inch baking pan covering the bottom and the sides
3. In a bowl, mix the dark chocolate and butter, microwave for 30 seconds or melt the mixture on a double boiler
4. In the meantime, combine the almond flour, sweetener, cocoa powder, and baking powder in a bowl
5. In a big bowl, beat the eggs with a mixer, then add in the butter and chocolate mixture and continue mixing
6. Slowly mix in the dry ingredients, until the mixture turns into a brownie batter consistency
7. Transfer the batter to the baking pan
8. Bake for 25-20 minutes, depending on the oven the baking time may vary, make sure you don't overbake them and the center is slightly moist to the touch
9. Allow the brownies to cool
10. Cut and serve!

Macros Per Serving – Calories:250 |Total Fat: 24g | Protein: 5g| **Net Carbs: 1g**

Smoothies

Micro-nutrient Greens Matcha Smoothie

Get a dose of your recommended greens with this micronutrient greens matcha smoothie!

Total Time: 5 Minutes

Serves: 1

Ingredients:
- 1 scoop Keto micro greens
- 2 tbsp collagen peptides
- 1 scoop MCT oil powder
- 1 tsp matcha powder
- ¼ cup full fat canned coconut milk
- ¼ cup frozen wild blackberries
- ½ cup of ice
- 1 cup of water
- 5 drops liquid stevia

Directions:
1. Add the micro greens, MCT oil powder, matcha powder, coconut milk, blackberries, ice, water, and stevia into the blender
2. Blend on high until smooth
3. Add in the collagen and pulse to combine
4. Enjoy!

Macros Per Serving – Calories:305 |Total Fat: 18g | Protein: 19g| **Net Carbs: 1g**

Mocha Smoothie

You can't go wrong with this Mocha Smoothie! It makes for a quick, satisfying, and tasty breakfast on-the-go!

Total Time: 5 Minutes

Serves: 3

Ingredients:
- ½ cup coconut milk and the thick cream from a can
- 1 ½ cup unsweetened almond milk
- 1 tsp vanilla extract
- 3 tbsp granulated stevia/erythritol blend
- 2 tsp instant coffee crystals, regular of decaffeinated
- 3 tbsp unsweetened cocoa powder
- 1 avocado, cut in half, pit removed

Directions:
1. Add the coconut milk, almond milk, vanilla extract, sweetener, coffee crystals, and cocoa powder to the blender
2. Blend until smooth
3. Add the avocado into the mixture, blend until smooth
4. Serve!

Macros Per Serving – Calories:176 |Total Fat: 6g | Protein: 3g| **Net Carbs: 4g**

Raspberry Coconut Smoothie

Get a taste of the islands with a hint of raspberry with this yummy smoothie!

Total Time: 5 Minutes

Serves: 2

Ingredients:
- 1 cup raspberry
- 1 cup coconut milk
- ½ tsp vanilla extract
- 1 pot of coconut yogurt
- Stevia, to taste

Directions:
1. Add the coconut yogurt, raspberry, coconut milk, vanilla extract, and stevia into the blender
2. Blend until smooth
3. Serve!

Macros Per Serving – Calories:554 |Total Fat: 49g | Protein: 8g| **Net Carbs: 9g**

Frosted Vanilla Blackberry Lemonade Smoothie

Frosted Vanilla Blackberry Lemonade is a refreshing treat you can enjoy anytime of the week!

Total Time: 5 Minutes
Serves: 2

Ingredients:
- 2/3 cup unsweetened almond or cashew milk
- ¼ cup lemon juice
- 1 tbsp collagen
- ½ tbsp stevia extract or 2 drops of stevia extract
- 2 pinches Himalayan salt or mineral salt
- 1 tsp vanilla extract
- ½ tsp glucomannan
- ½ cup blackberries, fresh or frozen
- 3 cups ice cubes, about one full tray

Directions:
1. Add in the lemon juice, almond milk, collagen, stevia, salt, and vanilla in blender
2. Mix on low for a few seconds
3. While the blender is on low, slowly add in glucomannan, blend on low for 30 more seconds and then turn if off
4. Add in blackberries and ice cubes, blend on high until completely blended
5. Enjoy!

Recipe Notes – Depending on how sweet your blackberries are, you may need to add more sweetener.

Macros Per Serving – Calories:136 |Total Fat: 2.2g | Protein: 2g| **Net Carbs: 2g**

Chocolate Berry Smoothie

Switch up your breakfast menu with this chocolate berry truffle smoothie! It's thick and rich like a milkshake, and tastes amazing!

Total Time: 5 Minutes

Serves: 2

Ingredients:
- ¾ cup frozen mixed berries (raspberries, black berries, and strawberries)
- ½ medium-sized hass avocado
- 2 tbsp pecans almonds
- 1 ½ tbsp unsweetened cocoa powder
- 2 (1g) packets stevia/erythritol blend
- 1 pinch salt
- ¾ tsp pure vanilla extract
- ¼ cup heavy whipping cream
- ½ cup water
- ¾ cup ice cubes

Directions:
1. Add in the frozen berries, avocado, pecan almond, cocoa powder, stevia/erythritol blend packets, salt, vanilla, heavy w all ingredients except the ice to a high-speed blender and process until smooth
2. Add the ice and pulse until smooth
3. Transfer to a glass and add toppings if desired
4. Serve immediately

Macros Per Serving – Calories:294 |Total Fat: 26g | Protein: 3g| **Net Carbs: 2g**

Strawberry Black Currant Smoothie

You'll love the healthy mix of strawberry and black currant in this creamy smoothie!

Total Time: 5 Minutes

Serves: 1

Ingredients:
- ½ cup black currants, fresh or frozen
- ¼ cup strawberries, 2-3 strawberries, fresh or frozen
- ¼ cup coconut milk or heavy whipping cream
- ½ cup water
- 2 tbsp chia seeds, whole or powdered
- ½ vanilla bean or ½ tsp sugar free vanilla extract

Optional:
- 5-7 drops liquid stevia extract

Directions:
1. Place the black currants, strawberries, coconut milk, water, chia seeds, and vanilla extract into a blender and pulse until smooth
2. Allow to sit for 2-5 minutes
3. Enjoy!

Recipe Note: You can also use raspberries or blackberries! If you're feeling hungry add a scoop (¼ cup) of vanilla or plain whey protein or egg white protein powder.

Macros Per Serving – Calories:228 |Total Fat: 17g | Protein: 5g| **Net Carbs: 8g**

Minty Green Protein Smoothie Shake

Dairy free and low in carbs, this Minty Green Protein Smoothie is the perfect way to start the day!

Total Time: 5 Minutes

Serves: 1

Ingredients:
- ½ avocado
- 1 cup fresh spinach
- 10-12 drops liquid stevia peppermint sweet drops
- 1 scoop whey protein (can be substituted for a dairy-free protein powder)
- ½ cup unsweetened almond milk
- ¼ tsp peppermint extract
- 1 cup ice

Optional:
- Cacao nibs

Directions:
1. Add the avocado, spinach, protein powder, and milk in a blender and blend until smooth
2. Add in the liquid stevia peppermint sweet drops, extract, and ice, and blend until thick
3. Taste and adjust stevia, as needed
4. Sprinkle the optional cacao nibs on top
5. Enjoy!

Macros Per Serving – Calories:293 |Total Fat: 15g | Protein: 28g| **Net Carbs: 4g**

Turmeric "Golden" Milkshake Turmeric

Just the perfect healthy drink. You can enjoy this keto turmeric milkshake both hot or cold!

Total Time: 5 Minutes

Serves: 1

Ingredients:
- ½L nondairy milk
- 2 tbsp coconut oil
- ½ tsp ginger powder
- ¼ tsp cinnamon
- ¾ tsp turmeric powder
- ¼ tsp vanilla
- Liquid stevia, to taste
- Pinch of himalayan salt
- 2 ice cubes

Directions:
1. Add in the nondairy milk, coconut oil, ginger powder, cinnamon, turmeric powder, vanilla, sweetener, pinch of salt, and ice cube in a high-powered blender
2. Blend on high for 30 seconds, or until thick and golden
3. Pour the shake into a glass
4. Sprinkle with cinnamon and turmeric

Recipe Notes - If your blender is not high powered, grate or mince the turmeric and ginger roots before adding it to the blender, or use powdered turmeric and ginger instead

Macros Per Serving – Calories:315 |Total Fat: 35g | Protein: 1g| **Net Carbs: 5g**

Chocolate Coconut Smoothie

Chocolate and coconut are such a great combo, you can enjoy any time of day with this smoothie!

Total Time: 5 Minutes

Serves: 1

Ingredients:
- ½ large avocado
- 1 ¼ cup almond milk
- ¼ cup coconut cream
- 1 tbsp flax meal or chia seeds
- 1 ½ tbsp cacao powder
- 1 tsp virgin coconut oil or MCT oil
- 1 tbsp almond butter or other nut seed butter

Optional:
- Water, to thin the smoothie if it's too thick

Topping:
- Whipped cream
- Cocoa nibs or chopped dark chocolate

Directions:
1. Add in the avocado, almond milk, coconut cream, flax meal or chia seeds, cacao powder, coconut oil or MCT oil, and almond butter or sub in the blender, blend until smooth
2. Pour into a glass and serve
3. Enjoy!

Macros Per Serving – Calories:510 |Total Fat: 42g | Protein: 12g| **Net Carbs: 6.8g**

Breakfast

Brie and Berries Crepe Breakfast

Something about the combination of fresh, sweet and juicy berries and creamy brie that makes this crepe breakfast work!

Prep Time: 5 Minutes
Cook Time: 15 Minutes
Total Time: 20 Minutes
Serves: 4

Ingredients:

Crepe batter:
- 4 oz. cream cheese
- 4 large eggs
- ½ tsp baking soda
- ¼ tsp sea salt

Toppings:
- 2 oz. chopped pecans
- 1 tbsp unsalted butter
- ¼ tsp cinnamon
- 4 oz. brie cheese, room temp
- Fresh mint leaves, for garnish

Directions:

1. Blend the batter ingredients – cream cheese eggs, baking soda and sea salt into a magic bullet or blender and blending until smooth
2. Place a non-stick pan over medium heat, add the unsalted butter
3. Once heated, ladle some of the crepe batter into the pan and swirl until the batter is thin and spread out evenly
4. Allow to cook until the top looks dry, about 2-3 minutes, then flip gently with a large spatula and cook the other side for a few seconds.
5. Repeat until you have about 12 crepes, layer them on top of each other on a plate while you prep the toppings/fillings
6. In a small pan, melt a tbsp of butter and toast the chopped pecans until fragrant, making sure they don't become too brown
7. Sprinkle with cinnamon and mix well, then transfer to a plate to cool
8. Slice the brie cheese.
9. Arrange the berries and brie on 1 crepe and top with some of the toasted pecans
10. Repeat with all the crepes
11. Garnish with the mint and enjoy rolled up or with a fork and knife!

Macros Per Serving – Calories:411 |Total Fat: 37g | Protein: 14g| **Net Carbs: 2g**

California Chicken Omelet

Combine the freshest ingredients – bacon, tomato, avocado and chicken - to make this amazing protein packed California Chicken Omelet!

Prep Time: 10 Minutes
Cook Time: 10 Minutes
Total Time: 20 Minutes
Serves 1

Ingredients:
- 4 eggs
- 4 slices bacon, cooked and chopped
- 2 oz. deli cut chicken
- ½ avocado
- 2 campari tomato
- 2 tbsp mayo
- 2 tsp mustard

Directions:
1. Place a nonstick pan over medium heat
2. In a small bowl, beat 2 eggs add them to a hot pan, pulling the sides of the eggs towards the center to cook the omelet
3. Season the omelet with salt and pepper
4. Once the eggs are halfway cooked about 5 minutes, add the deli cut chicken, bacon, sliced avocado and tomato along with a tablespoon of mayo and mustard to one half
5. Fold the omelet over onto itself and cover with a lid, cook for an additional 5 minutes
6. Enjoy!

Macros Per Serving – Calories:415 |Total Fat: 32g | Protein: 25g| **Net Carbs: 4g**

Cream Cheese Pancakes

Made without sugar and all rolled up, these delicious low carb cream cheese pancakes taste just like fried cheesecakes!

Prep Time: 3 Minutes
Cook Time: 9 Minutes
Total Time: 12 Minutes
Serves: 1

Ingredients:
- 2 oz. cream cheese
- 2 eggs
- 1 tsp granulated sugar substitute
- ½ tsp cinnamon

Directions:
1. Place the cream cheese, eggs, sugar sub, and cinnamon into a blender or magic blends, blend until smooth
2. Allow to rest for 2 minutes to settle the bubbles
3. Place a pan greased with butter or pam spray over medium heat, once heated pour ¼ of the batter into the pan
4. Cook for 2 minutes or until golden brown, flip and cook 1 minute on the other side
5. Repeat until the batter is gone
6. Serve with fresh berries and sugar free syrup

Macros Per Serving 4 pancakes – Calories:344 |Total Fat: 29g | Protein: 17g| **Net Carbs: 1g**

Mexican Frittata

All jazzed up with a Mexican flair, this omelet is filled with a seasoned beef, salsa, chopped veggies, all top with cheddar cheese!

Prep Time: 10 Minutes
Cook Time: 20 Minutes
Total Time: 30 Minutes
Serves: 6

Ingredients:
- 8 eggs, beaten
- 1 tbsp olive oil
- ½ lb ground beef
- 2 tsp taco seasoning
- ½ cup salsa
- 1 small green pepper chopped
- 1/3 lb plum tomatoes, sliced
- 3 scallions, chopped
- ¼ tsp salt
- ½ cup grated cheddar cheese

Directions:
1. Preheat the oven to 375 degrees F
2. Place a medium skillet over medium heat, brown the ground beef in the olive oil
3. Add in the taco seasoning and salsa, stir to coat evenly, then remove the seasoned meat from the skillet
4. Add the green pepper to the skillet, cook for a few minutes, until crispy
5. Add the meat back to the skillet with the tomato and scallions
6. Add in the beaten eggs on top, and sprinkle with the salt and cheese
7. Bake for 20 to 25 minutes, or until the frittata has set and is no longer jiggly
8. Allow the frittata to cool before cutting
9. Serve!

Macros Per Serving – Calories:229 |Total Fat: 15g | Protein: 18g| **Net Carbs: 1g**

Raspberry & Cream Crepes

Raspberry and cream cheese go together so well, and are even better when they're inside of a light crepe!

Prep Time: 10 Minutes
Cook Time: 30 Minutes
Total Time: 40 Minutes
Serves 2
Yields 6 crepes

Ingredients:

Crepe Batter:
- 2 large eggs
- 2 oz. cream cheese
- 10 drops liquid stevia
- ¼ tsp cinnamon
- ¼ tsp baking soda
- 1/8 tsp sea salt

Filling:
- ½ cup raspberry
- 4 oz. cream cheese
- ½ tsp vanilla extract
- 2 tbsp powdered erythritol

Directions:
1. In a bowl, combine the cream cheese and eggs and beat them with an electric hand mixer until smooth
2. Add in the stevia, cinnamon, baking soda and sea salt, combine well
3. In a nonstick pan over medium heat, add in the butter or coconut oil to lightly grease the pan
4. Once heated, pour in about ¼ cup of batter while swirling the pan to gently spread it the edges
5. Cook until the edges begin to crisp about 3 minutes per crepe
6. Loosen the edges with a spatula and then gently flip the crepe, repeat until all the batter is gone
7. Prepare the filling by combining the cream cheese, vanilla extract and powdered erythritol in a small bowl, then beat with an electric hand mixer until smooth and creamy
8. Add a small amount of the filling to the center of each crepe
9. Add some fresh raspberry and wrap up the crepe
10. Enjoy with extra cinnamon!

Macros Per Serving of 3 Crepes with Filling – Calories: 390 |Total Fat: 32g | Protein: 13g|**Net Carbs: 7g**

Cauliflower Hash Browns

Rich and buttery, these low-carb hash browns will totally wow any hash brown fan!

Prep Time: 10 Minutes
Cook Time: 20 Minutes
Total Time: 30 Minutes
Serves: 4

Ingredients:
- 15 oz. cauliflower, rinsed, trimmed and grated
- 3 eggs
- ½ yellow onion, grated
- 1 tsp salt
- 2 pinches pepper
- 4 oz. butter or oil, for frying

Directions:
1. Rinse, trim and grate the cauliflower using a grater or food processor
2. Transfer the cauliflower to a large bowl, add in the eggs, yellow onion, salt, and pepper, mix well and then set aside for 5 to 10 minutes
3. In a large skillet over medium heat, melt the butter or add the oil
4. Working in batches of 3-4 hash browns, scoop of the grated cauliflower mixture in the frying pan and flatten them carefully until they're about 3–4 inches in diameter
5. Fry for 4 to 5 minutes on each side, make sure to adjust the heat so they don't burn and don't flip the hash browns too soon

Recipe Notes: Keep the first batch warm in the oven as you cook the other batches

Macros Per Serving – Calories:278 | Total Fat: 26g | Protein: 7g| **Net Carbs: 5g**

Shakshuka – Eggs Poached in Tomato Sauce

Shakshuka is a delicious traditional Middle Eastern dish which is made with creamy eggs poached in a flavorful tomato sauce. It's low in carbs and will be ready in under 30 minutes!

Prep Time:10 Minutes
Cook Time: 10 Minutes
Total Time: 20 Minutes
Serves 2

Ingredients:
- 2 cups marinara sauce
- 2 chili pepper
- 8 eggs
- 2 oz. feta cheese
- ¼ tbps cumin
- Salt, to taste
- Pepper, to taste
- Fresh basil, as garnish

Directions:
1. Preheat the oven to 400 degrees F
2. Place a small skillet over medium heat, add a cup of the marinara sauce and some of the chopped chili pepper
3. Allow the chili pepper to cook for about 5 minutes in the sauce
4. Crack and gently lower the eggs into the marinara sauce
5. Sprinkle feta cheese all over the eggs and then season with the salt, pepper and cumin
6. Using an oven mitt, place the skillet into the oven and bake for about 10 minutes
7. Once the eggs are cooked, but still runny, remove the skillet out with an oven mitt
8. Chop the fresh basil and sprinkle it over the shakshuka
9. Enjoy!

Macros Per Serving – Calories:490 |Total Fat: 34g | Protein: 35g| **Net Carbs: 4g**

Chia Berry Yogurt Parfaits

Fall in love with this healthy parfait that's made with a chia pudding, berry layers, and topped with a coconut crumble!

Prep Time: 10 Minutes
Refrigerate Time: 30 Minutes
Total Time: 40 Minutes
Serves: 4

Ingredients:
For the chia pudding:
- ⅓ cup chia seeds
- ¼ tsp vanilla bean powder or ½ tsp sugar free vanilla extract
- ¼ tsp ground cinnamon
- ⅔ cup water
- ½ cup coconut cream
- 1 tbsp powdered erythritol or swerve or 2-3 drops of stevia

For berry and yogurt layer:
- 1 cup mixed frozen berries
- 1 cup full fat greek or coconut yogurt or cream

For coconut and seed crumble:
- ⅓ cup flaked coconut, preferably toasted
- 2 tbsp sunflower seeds
- 2 tbsp pumpkin seeds

Directions:
1. Prepare the chia pudding layer by combining the chia seeds, vanilla bean powders, ground cinnamon, water coconut cream and erythritol, allow to sit for at least 30 minutes or overnight
2. Defrost and crush the berries together with a fork to form a paste
3. In a small bowl, mix together the flaked coconuts, sunflower seeds, and pumpkin seeds
4. Prepare the parfaits by layering the chia pudding, crumble, crushed berries, and yogurt

Recipe Notes: You can also make the parfaits in advance without the crumble and add the crumble topping before serving.

Macros Per Serving – Calories:319 |Total Fat: 25g | Protein: 21g| **Net Carbs: 7g**

Filipino Breakfast Torta Omelet

This hearty Filipino breakfast torta is so easy to make and a great for a quick breakfast!

Prep Time: 10 Minutes
Cook Time: 20 Minutes
Total Time: 30 Minutes
Serves: 4

Ingredients:
- 1/3 cup chopped onions
- 2 large garlic cloves, minced
- 1 lb ground beef or pork
- 1 tbsp fish or soy sauce
- ½ tsp salt
- ¼ tsp freshly ground black pepper
- 6 large eggs beaten
- 2 tbsp oil, divided
- 2 green onions, thinly sliced

Directions:
1. In a large skillet over medium heat, add 2 tbsp of the oil
2. Once heated, add onions and garlic and sauté, stirring often, until translucent, about 5 minutes Then add the ground beef or pork, cook until cooked through, about 8 to 10 minutes, stirring often and break the large clumps up with a wooden spoon, season with salt and pepper
3. Drain the beef mixture and allow it to cool for 10 minutes
4. Add in the eggs and fish or soy sauce to the cooled beef mixture, stir to combine
5. In an 8-inch non-stick skillet over medium-low heat, add 1 tsp of oil
6. Once heated, ladle a scoop of the mixture, about ¼ into the hot oil
7. Allow the omelet to set for 3 minutes, then sprinkle with the green onions, flip the omelet and cook 2 more minutes, then transfer to a plate
8. Repeat with remaining oil, egg-beef mixture, and green onions until the mixture is gone.
9. Serve the omelet individually, or stacked with chili sauce

Macros Per Serving – Calories:456 |Total Fat: 36g | Protein: 28g| **Net Carbs: 1g**

Breakfast "Crunch" Cereal

Miss the crunch of cereal? Enjoy this keto cereal recipe that's made with a mix of seeds, nuts and coconut!

Prep Time: 5 Minutes
Cook Time: 40 Minutes
Total Time: 45 Minutes
Serves: 12

Ingredients:
- 1 cup of unsweetened shredded coconut
- 1 cup of unsweetened coconut flakes
- ½ cup of flaked almonds
- ½ cup of flaxseeds
- 1/3 cup of pepitas
- 1/3 cup of chia seeds
- 1/3 cup of sunflower seeds
- 1 tbsp of cinnamon, ground
- 1/3 cup of erythritol
- 1/3 cup of coconut oil, melted
- 1 tsp of vanilla extract

Directions:
1. Preheat oven to 300 degrees F
2. In a bowl, mix together the shredded coconut, coconut flakes, almond flakes, flaxseeds, pepitas, chia seeds, sunflower seeds, cinnamon, erythritol, coconut oil, and vanilla extract, combine well
3. Spread evenly over a lined cookie sheet
4. Bake for 25 to 35 minutes, making sure to stir every 5 minutes to prevent burning
5. Remove from the oven when the ingredients are golden brown and toasted
6. Allow the cereal to cool completely before storing in an airtight container
7. Enjoy

Macros Per Serving – Calories:244|Total Fat: 22g | Protein: 4g| **Net Carbs: 3g**

Greek Spinach, Herb and Feta Wrap

Indulge in this Greek wrap that's made with fluffy eggs and filled with spinach, herbs and feta!

Prep Time: 10 Minutes
Cook Time: 15 Minutes
Total Time: 25 Minutes
Serves: 2

Ingredients:
- 5 whole eggs
- 3 egg whites
- 1 tsp sesame oil
- ½ tsp salt
- 2 cups spinach leaves
- ½ cup crumbled feta
- 4 leaves basil, roughly chopped
- 3 whole sun-dried tomatoes, chopped

Optional:
- 1 tsp olive oil

Directions:
1. In a large mixing bowl, combine the whole eggs, egg whites, salt, and sesame oil, whisk together until the mixture is semi - foamy, about :30 to 1 minutes
2. Spray a non-stick pan with cooking spray, place over medium heat, pour half of the egg mixture into the skillet, cover and then reduce the heat to medium-low
3. Once cooked through, remove from the pan and allow to cool
4. Prepare the second wrap in the same way, cooking medium-low and slowly
5. Then prepare the filling by placing the spinach in the skillet on low heat, cook until the spinach is gently wilted the leaves
6. Divide the feta, sun-dried tomatoes, basil, and oil, and prepare to fill the wraps
7. Start with a layer of wilted spinach, followed with the feta, basil, and a drizzle of oil
8. Roll from one end to the other and enjoy!

Macros Per Serving – Calories:361 |Total Fat: 25g | Protein: 27g| **Net Carbs: 4g**

Smoked Salmon Breakfast Salad

A salad for breakfast? Absolutely! All fresh and packed with protein, this your personalized breakfast salad will be ready in no time.

Total Time: 15 Minutes

Serves: 1

Ingredients:
- 2 cups of butter lettuce or chopped salad of your choice
- 1 filet of smoked salmon
- Chopped/grated raw vegetables of your choice, cucumbers, carrots, bell peppers, snap peas, cabbage, avocado
- Fresh herbs or seasoning blends
- Dressing, squirt of lemon/lime, vinegar & olive oil or prepared salad dressing of your choice
- Extra toppings, sunflower seeds, pepitas, shredded cheese, nuts of your choice

Directions:
1. Place the bed of lettuce in a bowl
2. Top with the salmon, raw veggies of your choice, herbs or seasoning blend
3. Then add a drizzle of dressing or squirt of lime/lemon juice, toss
4. Add the extra topping of your choice
5. Enjoy!

Macros Per Serving will vary on your ingredients

Breakfast Sausage with Guacamole Stacks

Your favorite breakfast ingredients – avocado, eggs and sausage, are all stacked and ready to go with this easy Sausage & Guac recipe!

Prep Time: 10 Minutes
Cook Time: 15 Minutes
Total Time: 25 Minutes
Serves 2

Ingredients:

Quick Guacamole:
- 1 medium avocado
- ½ small white or yellow onion, chopped
- 2 tbsp fresh lime juice
- Salt, to taste
- Pepper, to taste

Stacks:
- 1-2 tbsp ghee, for frying
- 170g Italian sausage meat
- 2 large eggs
- Salt, to taste
- Pepper, to taste

Directions:
1. Prepare the guacamole by cutting the avocado in half and scooping it into a bowl
2. Add the lime juice, onion, salt and pepper, then mash with a fork and set aside
3. Create small patties with the sausage meat, wash hands and then set aside
4. Greased a pan with half of the ghee and then place it over medium heat
5. Once heated, add the sausage to the pan and cook for 2-3 minutes, then flip on the other side and cook for 1-2 more minutes, set aside
6. Grease the pan with the remaining ghee and crack in the eggs, cook until the egg whites are cooked through and the egg yolks are still runny - If you use an egg mold then lower the heat since it will take longer to cook through
7. Once done, top each patty with the prepared guacamole and the fried egg
8. Season with salt and pepper to taste
9. Enjoy!

Macros Per Serving – Calories:509 |Total Fat: 43.9g | Protein: 20.1g| **Net Carbs: 4.4g**

Egg Crust Breakfast Pizza

If you love left over pizza for breakfast, then you'll love this Low-Carb alternative! Made with yummy egg-crust, this breakfast pizza is topped with all your favorite toppings!

Prep Time: 10 Minutes
Cook Time: 10 Minutes
Total Time: 20 Minutes
Serves: 1-2

Ingredients:
- 1-2 tsp olive oil
- 2 eggs
- 4-5 small grape tomatoes, thinly sliced
- 6 slices of pepperoni, cut in half to make half-moon pieces
- 6-8 black olives, thinly sliced
- 1 oz mozzarella, cut into small cubes
- Italian Seasoning of your choice, to taste
- Dried oregano, to taste

Directions:
1. Preheat the oven broil
2. In a bowl, beat the eggs
3. Slice tomatoes and olives, cut pepperoni in half, and cut mozzarella into small cubes
4. In a small pan over medium heat, add the olive oil
5. Once heated, add the eggs, season of choic and oregano, and cook until eggs start to set on the bottom, about 2 minutes.
6. Sprinkle on half each of the tomatoes, pepperoni, olives, and mozzarella, followed by a second layer with half of each -add plenty of cheese on top
7. Cover the pan and all the eggs to cook until mostly set and cheese starts to melt, about 3-4 minutes.
8. Then place the pan under the broil and cook until the cheese is melted and the top is golden brown, about 2-3 minutes
9. Serve!

Macros Per Serving – Calories:325 |Total Fat: 23g | Protein: 24g| **Net Carbs: 3g**

Cheesy Italian Omelet

Filled with basil, mozzarella cheese and your favorite cold cut, you'll look forward to making this delicious low carb omelet in the morning!

Prep Time: 5 Minutes
Cook Time: 3 Minutes
Total Time: 8 Minutes
Serves: 1

Ingredients:
- 2 eggs
- 1 tbsp water
- 1 tbsp butter
- 3 thin slices deli Sopressata (you can sub in salami or prosciutto if that's what you have)
- 6 fresh basil leaves
- 5 thin slices fresh, ripe tomato
- 2 oz fresh mozzarella cheese
- Salt, to taste
- Pepper, to taste

Directions:
1. In a bowl, whisk together the eggs and water
2. In a non-stick pan over medium low heat, melt the butter
3. Once heated, pour in the egg mixture and cook for 30 seconds
4. Spread the meat slices on one half of the egg mixture
5. Top with the cheese, tomatoes, and basil slices, then season with salt and pepper
6. Cook for about 2 minutes or until the empty side of the egg has set
7. Then use a spatula to gently fold the omelet in half
8. Cover the pan and cook on low heat for 1-2 minutes or until the omelet is cooked through
9. Remove the omelet by tilting the pan and sliding the omelet gently out onto a plate

Macros Per Serving – Calories:451 |Total Fat: 36g | Protein: 33g| **Net Carbs: 3g**

Lunch

Asian Cashew Chicken Lettuce Wraps

Perfect as a quick lunch, these cashew chicken lettuce wraps are low in carbs and calories!

Prep Time: 15 Minutes
Cook Time: 8 Minutes
Total Time: 23 Minutes
Serves: 8

Ingredients:
- 1 lb boneless, skinless chicken breasts cut into bite sized pieces
- 4 tbsp oyster sauce
- 4 tbsp low-sodium soy sauce
- 2 tbsp sesame oil or olive oil
- 2 cloves garlic minced or grated
- 1 tsp grated fresh ginger
- 1 tsp chili paste
- 1/3 cup raw cashews
- 8 Boston lettuce leaves

Toppings:
- Thinly-sliced basil
- Sesame seeds

Directions:
1. Place the chicken in a ziplock bag with the chili paste, oyster sauce, and soy sauce
2. Allow the chicken marinate for 10 minutes
3. Place a large skillet over medium heat, add 1 tbsp of garlic, sesame oil, ginger, and cook for 30 seconds or until fragrant
4. Turn the heat up to medium high, add the chicken and the remaining oil, and stir-fry until cooked through, about 5 minutes
5. Once cooked, add the cashews and cook for another 1-2 minutes.
6. Spoon the mixture into the individual lettuce leaves, top with basil and sesame seeds
7. Enjoy!

Macros Per Serving 2 lettuce cups – Calories:165 |Total Fat: 8g | Protein: 17g| **Net Carbs: 0.1g**

Zucchini Crust Grilled Cheese

No bread, no problem with this easy recipe! You'll replace it with low carb zucchini to enjoy the same bit of crunch with a gooey center.

Prep Time: 5 Minutes
Cook Time: 40 Minutes
Total Time: 45 Minutes
Serves: 2

Ingredients:

For the zucchini crust slices:
- 4 cups shredded zucchini
- 1 egg
- ½ cup shredded mozzarella cheese
- 4 tbsp grated Parmesan cheese
- 1 tsp dried oregano
- ½ tsp salt
- Pinch of ground black pepper

For the grilled cheese:
- 1 tbsp butter, room temperature
- ⅓ cup /3 oz /85g sharp cheddar cheese, grated/shredded, at room temperature

Directions:
1. Preheat oven to 450 degrees F and place a rack in the middle.
2. Line a baking sheet with parchment paper and liberally grease it, set aside
3. Place the shredded zucchini in a microwave-safe dish, microwave on high for 6 minutes
4. Transfer to a dishcloth or a tea towel, twist and squeeze as much moisture as you can since the zucchini has to be dry to be crisp
5. In a bowl, mix the zucchini, egg, mozzarella cheese, Parmesan cheese, oregano, salt, and pepper
6. Spread the zucchini mixture onto the lined baking sheet, shape into 4 squares
7. Bake for 15 to 20 minutes or until lightly golden brown
8. Remove from the oven and allow it to cool 10 minutes before removing them off the parchment paper
9. Place a skillet over medium heat and butter the top side of each slice of zucchini crust bread, place the one slice of bread in the pan, buttered side down, and sprinkle with the cheese
10. Too with the remaining slice of zucchini crust bread, buttered side up
11. Turn the heat down a little and cook until golden brown, about 2 to 4 minutes
12. Gently flip and cook until golden brown on the other side, about 2 to 4 minutes
13. Enjoy

Macros Per Serving – Calories:174 |Total Fat: 10g | Protein: 15g| **Net Carbs: 3g**

Poke with Ahi Tuna and Citrus

The easiest keto-friendly poke you've ever had! Made with Ahi Tuna and a splash of citrus flavors, you'll love having it for lunch.

Total Time: 15 Minutes

Serves: 2

Ingredients:
- 8 oz Yellowfin tuna (Ahi tuna) fillet
- 1 tbsp coconut aminos
- 5 sprigs cilantro or Italian parsley (about 1/4 cup chopped)
- ½ hass avocado
- 2 tbsp sesame oil
- 1 tbsp sesame seeds
- ¼ cup pili nuts
- 1 tsp sea salt
- ¼ ruby red grapefruit

Directions:
1. Slice the ahi into ¼ inch cubes, place in a large bowl
2. Add in the coconut aminos, sesame oil and salt, gently toss
3. Cut the grapefruit in half and cut out the sections, add to the bowl
4. Mince the cilantro, add it to the bowl
5. Chop up the pili nuts, dice your avocado, add both into the bowl
6. Gently toss to combine
7. Divide the ahi mix between two bowls and garnish with sesame seeds
8. Enjoy!

Macros Per Serving – Calories:445 |Total Fat: 33g | Protein: 39g| **Net Carbs: 10g**

Chicken Quesadilla

You won't miss tortillas with this Cheesy & Chicken Quesadilla Recipe that features bell peppers, green onion and tomatoes.

Prep Time: 5 Minutes
Cook Time: 10 Minutes
Total Time: 15 Minutes
Serves: 1

Ingredients:
- 1 ½ cups mozzarella cheese
- 1 ½ cups cheddar cheese
- 1 cup cooked chicken
- ¼ cup bell pepper
- ¼ cup diced tomato
- ⅛ cup green onion

To Serve:
- Sour cream
- Salsa
- Guacamole
- Fresh basil, garnish
- Parsley, garnish
- Cilantro, garnish

Directions:
1. Preheat oven to 400 degrees F
2. Cover the pizza pan with Parchment Paper
3. In a bowl, mix together the cheese then evenly spread them over the parchment paper
4. Bake the cheese shell for 5 minutes
5. Pour off any extra oil as soon as it comes out of the oven
6. Place the cooked chicken over half of the cheese shell, add the sliced peppers, diced tomato and the chopped green onion on top
7. Fold the Cheese shell in half over the chicken and veggies, press it firmly, then return it to the oven for another 4 to 5 minutes
8. Serve with sour cream, salsa and guacamole
9. Garnish with chopped fresh basil, parsley or cilantro

Recipe Note: To reheat the quesadilla, preheat the oven to 400 degrees F and bake for 6-8 minutes (if cold)

Macros Per Serving – Calories:599 |Total Fat: 50g | Protein: 53g| **Net Carbs: 5g**

Mongolian Beef Bowl

This Mongolian beef bowl features beef covered in a savory garlic, ginger sauce. Just serve it up with steamed broccoli or cauliflower rice!

Prep Time: 10 Minutes
Cook Time: 15 Minutes
Total Time: 25 Minutes
Serves: 4

Ingredients:

- 1 lb flank steak sliced into bite-size stripes
- 2 tbsp olive oil, divided
- 1 tbsp fresh ginger, peeled and grated
- 2 garlic cloves minced
- 2 tbsp coconut aminos
- ½ cup water
- 1/3 cup So Nourished Erythritol
- 1 tsp red pepper flakes
- 1-2 tsp xanthan gum to thicken the sauce
- Salt, to taste
- Pepper, to taste
- 1 scallion sliced, for topping

Directions:

1. In a saucepan over medium heat, add half of olive oil
2. Once heated, add the minced garlic and grated ginger and fry for 30 seconds
3. Add the water, coconut aminos, erythritol, and red pepper flakes, simmer on high for 3 to 4 minutes
4. Remove from heat and set aside
5. Add in the xanthan gum and beef strips to a zip bag, toss well
6. In a frying pan, add the other half of olive oil
7. Once heated, add the beef strips and fry stirring until begin to get brown, set aside
8. Place a clean pan over medium heat (or use the pan with beef), add the beef and prepared sauce, a pinch of salt and pepper, cook for another minute stirring constantly
9. Divide the beef between plates and garnish with sliced scallions
10. Serve with steamed broccoli florets or cauliflower rice

Macros Per Serving – Calories:318 |Total Fat: 19g | Protein: 31g| **Net Carbs: 2g**

Quick Spicy Tuna Rolls

Spicy tuna rolls recipe will give you the right amount of crunch and heat! Plus, it's so fast and easy to make.

Total Time: 5 Minutes
Serves: 1

Ingredients:
- 1 cucumber
- 1 can or a pouch of tuna
- 1 tbsp mayo (for tuna mixture)
- 2 tsp sriracha
- 2 tsp garlic powder
- Salt, to taste
- Pepper, to taste
- Avocado, sliced and cut to match the width of cucumber strips

Sauce:
- 2 tbsp mayo
- 2 tsp sriracha

Directions:
1. Slice the cucumbers lengthwise with a vegetable peeler for thin strips
2. If needed, drain the tuna and mix with mayo, sriracha, garlic powder, salt and pepper, mixture should be slightly moist but not wet
3. Place the cucumber strips on prep surface and spread the tuna mixture tightly along leaving about 1 inch at the end of the strip
4. Place the avocado pieces at the end of cucumber strip on top of tuna and tightly roll
5. Prepare the sauce by mixing together the mayo and sriracha in a bowl, then drizzle over cucumber rolls

Macros Per Serving – Calories:701 |Total Fat: 50g | Protein: 39g| **Net Carbs: 7g**

Buddha Bowl

What's a Buddha bowl? It's a whole lot of healthy and delicious ingredients mixed together to make the perfect lunch!

Prep Time: 5 Minutes
Cook Time: 10 Minutes
Total Time: 15 Minutes
Serves: 1

Ingredients:
- 1 bag frozen cauliflower, seasoned with salt and pepper and oil (optional)
- ½ avocado
- ½ tbsp olive oil
- 1 tsp soy sauce
- 1 oz mushrooms
- 3 oz spinach
- Salt, to taste

Directions:
1. In a skillet over medium heat, add the oil and spinach, sauté for a few seconds until the spinach changes color and wilts, then set aside – be careful not to over cook
2. Sauté the chopped mushrooms in oil and soy sauce
3. Prep cauliflower by sautéing it with oil and spices
4. Once done, top with mushrooms, spinach and avocado
5. Enjoy!

Macros Per Serving – Calories:411 |Total Fat: 2g | Protein: 11g| **Net Carbs: 13g**

Fish Tacos

Celebrate Taco Tuesday by whipping up a batch of crunchy and flaky fish tacos with this 100% keto-friendly recipe!

Prep Time: 20 Minutes
Cook Time: 15 Minutes
Total Time: 35 Minutes
Serves 8

Ingredients:
- 8 oz firm white-flesh fish such as flounder or cod
- 1/3 cup sour cream or coconut cream with 2 tsp apple cider vinegar
- 2 tsp apple cider vinegar
- 4 cloves garlic, pressed
- kosher salt, to taste
- 1/2 cup whey protein isolate
- 1 tsp baking powder
- 1 ½ tsp chili powder
- ¼ - ½ tsp kosher salt, to taste
- 1 egg
- 1 tbsp sour cream or coconut cream
- 2 tsp apple cider vinegar
- coconut oil or cooking oil, of choice

For Serving:
- 1 batch keto-friendly grain-free tortillas
- 1 batch pico de gallo salsa
- Guacamole
- Limes

Directions:
1. In a bowl, mix the sour or coconut cream, vinegar, garlic and season to taste with salt
2. Prepare the fish by cutting the fish across the grain of the flesh into strips that are about 1/2 inch wide
3. Add the fish to the cream marinade, cover and refrigerate for two hours or preferably overnight
4. Place a skillet or pan over medium/low heat, add the oil about ½-inch deep
5. While the oil heats up, mix together the whey protein, baking powder, chili powder and salt in a shallow plate or dish, set aside
6. In a different place or dish whisk together the egg, cream and vinegar, set aside

7. Prepare the fish by lightly removing excess marinade, dip it in the egg mix, followed by the whey protein mix
8. Immediately placing it the hot oil and basting the top, frying it on both sides until deep golden and then transfer to a paper-lined plate for a couple minutes
9. Serve right away with the heated tortillas, plenty of limes and your salsa of choice!

Recipe Notes:

You can also make your own chili powder mix with 3/4 tsp paprika, 1/4 tsp garlic powder, 1/4 tsp onion powder, 1/4 tsp dried oregano, 1/8 tsp cayenne pepper and 1/8 tsp dried cumin.

Macros Per Serving (1 Fish Taco)– Calories:48 |Protein: 9g| **Net Carbs: 2g (from the keto-friendly tortilla)**

Creamy Butternut Squash Soup

Make this butternut squash soup recipe that is so comforting during fall and winter! It's made with coconut and super easy to create. .

Prep Time: 10 Minutes
Cook Time: 60 Minutes
Total Time: 1 H 10 Minutes
Serves: 8

Ingredients:
- 1 (2-lb) butternut squas, cut in half lengthwise, seeds removed
- 2 tbsp avocado oil, divided
- 6 cloves garlic, minced
- 2 tbsp fresh thyme
- ½ tsp cinnamon
- 1/8 tsp nutmeg
- 4 cup chicken bone broth, or any broth of choice
- 1 (13.5-oz) can coconut milk
- Sea salt, to taste
- Black pepper, to taste

Directions:
1. Preheat the oven to 400 degrees F
2. Line a baking sheet with foil or parchment paper
3. Place the butternut squash halves open side up onto the baking sheet, drizzle with a tbsp of avocado oil, then sprinkle with sea salt and black pepper
4. Flip over, face down and roast the butternut squash in the oven for about 40 to 55 minutes, until a knife can easily pierce the squash
5. Once the squash has roasted for 30 minutes, add the remaining tbsp of avocado oil in a large pot over medium heat
6. Once heated, add the minced garlic, cinnamon, nutmeg and thyme, sauté for about a minute, until fragrant
7. Add the broth and coconut milk, simmer for about 20 minutes, or until the squash is done
8. Scoop the squash out of the shells into the soup, then use an immersion blender to puree until smooth
9. Enjoy!

Macros Per Serving – Calories:183 |Total Fat: 12g | Protein: 6g| **Net Carbs: 10g**

Cobb Salad

This simple Cobb salad recipe features bacon, chicken breast slices, tomato and avocado, making it so perfect for lunch.

Prep Time: 10 Minutes
Cook Time: 5 Minutes
Total Time: 15 Minutes
Serves 1-2

Ingredients:
- 2 strips bacon
- 2 oz chicken breast
- ½ campari tomato
- ¼ avocado
- 1 cup spinach
- 1 hard-boiled egg
- ½ tsp white vinegar
- 1 tbsp olive oil

Directions:
1. Shred or slice the cook chicken, which ever one you prefer, set aside
2. Dice the tomato and avocado, set aside
3. Slice the hard-boiled egg, set aside
4. Place the spinach in a large mixing bowl
5. Top with the diced tomatoes, hard-boiled egg, avocado, chicken breast and bacon strips
6. Top with the oil and vinegar
7. Toss to combine and enjoy!

Macros Per Serving – Calories:600 |Total Fat: 48g | Protein: 43g| **Net Carbs: 3g**

Philly Cheesesteak Stuffed Peppers

Complete with roast beef, onions, and tender mushrooms, these easy to make Philly cheesesteak stuffed peppers will make lunch-time 100% better!

Prep Time: 10 Minutes
Cook Time: 30 Minutes
Total Time: 40 Minutes
Serves 2

Ingredients:
- 3 bell peppers, cut in half lengthwise, ribs and seeds removed
- 2 tbsp butter or bacon fat, divided
- 1 medium to large yellow onion, julienned
- 8 oz crimini mushrooms, sliced
- 2 lbs roast beef sandwich cuts into strips or 4 boxes (9 oz. each) beef steaks
- 4 cloves garlic, minced
- 1 tsp mineral salt
- ½ tsp cayenne pepper
- ¾ cup mozzarella, provolone, or pepper jack cheese, shredded, divided

Optional:
- ¼ tsp red pepper flakes

Directions:
1. Preheat the oven to 400-degree F
2. Grease a 9- by 13-inch dish
3. Then place the pepper halves in the dish and pre-bake for about 10 to 15 minutes, until soft
4. In the meanwhile, place skillet over medium-high heat and melt 1 tablespoon butter
5. Once heated, add the onions and mushrooms and sauté, stirring often, until the onions are translucent
6. Add the remaining butter, roast beef, garlic, salt, cayenne pepper, and red pepper flakes to the skillet Sauté for an additional 10 to 15 minutes, or until the onions are caramelized and meat is heated
7. Remove the peppers from the oven, add about 1 tbsp of cheese to the bottom of each pepper half
8. Stuff the peppers with the meat mixture, top with remaining cheese
9. Bake for 10 to 15 minutes, or until cheese is melted and they begin to lightly brown
10. Enjoy!

Macros Per Serving – Calories:302 |Total Fat: 13g | Protein: 37g| **Net Carbs: 5g**

Sri Lankan Spicy Chili Cabbage Stir Fry

If you're craving something light for lunch, try this spicy chili cabbage stirfry recipe that's flavorful and 100% vegetarian!

Prep Time: 10 Minutes
Cook Time: 10 Minutes
Total Time: 20 Minutes
Serves: 4

Ingredients:
- Half a head of cabbage
- 1-2 garlic pods
- 1 large onion
- Sprig of curry leaves
- Pinch of turmeric powder
- ½ tsp of red chili flecks
- 2-3 tbsp of oil
- ½ lime

Directions:
1. Slice the cabbage, onion, garlic and set aside
2. Place a non-stick skillet over low heat, sauté the cabbage until they wilt and there is no moisture left in the skillet
3. Once the moisture has evaporated from cabbage, keep the heat low and pour in the oil, add the sliced onions, curry leaves, garlic and a pinch of turmeric powder and salt to taste
4. Cook for 5 minutes, or until the cabbage edges are slightly burn, then remove from heat
5. Add in the chili flecks and mix it into the cabbage stir-fry.
6. Taste and season with salt if necessary, and add a drizzle a bit of lime juice and mix
7. Serve warm over cauliflower rice or with the main dish of your choice

Macros Per Serving – Calories:639 |Total Fat: g | Protein: 29g| **Net Carbs: 8g**

Chicken Enchilada Bowl

This Mexican favorite is now keto-friendly with this recipe! It's so easy to make, filling and ridiculously yummy!

Prep Time: 20 Minutes
Cook Time: 30 Minutes
Total Time: 50 Minutes
Serves: 4

Ingredients:

- 2 tbsp coconut oil (for searing chicken)
- 1 lb of boneless, skinless chicken thighs
- ¾ cup red enchilada sauce
- ¼ cup water
- ¼ cup chopped onion
- 1 (4 oz) can diced green chiles

For toppings:

- 1 whole avocado, diced
- 1 cup shredded cheese, mild cheddar cheese
- ¼ cup chopped pickled jalapenos
- ½ cup sour cream
- 1 roma tomato, chopped

Directions:

1. In a pot or dutch oven over medium heat, add the coconut oil
2. Once heat, sear chicken thighs until lightly brown
3. Add in the enchilada sauce and water, then add in the onion and green chiles, reduce the heat to a simmer and cover. Cook the chicken for 17 to 25 minutes or until chicken is fully cooked and tender
4. Carefully remove the chicken and transfer to a plate
5. Chop or shred the chicken, then add it back into the pot
6. Allow the chicken simmer uncovered for an additional 10 minutes to absorb flavor and the sauce to reduce
7. Transfer to a bowl and top with avocado, cheese, jalapeno, sour cream, tomato, and other desired toppings
8. Enjoy alone or over cauliflower rice if desired!

Macros Per Serving – Calories:568 |Total Fat: 40g | Protein: 38g| **Net Carbs: 6g**

Zucchini Noodles with Garlic Shrimp

Combine Zucchini noodles with garlic shrimp and you can enjoy a deliciously healthy meal in about 20 minutes!

Prep Time: 15 Minutes
Cook Time: 6 Minutes
Total Time: 21 Minutes
Serves 4

Ingredients:

- 6 zucchinis, washed
- 1 lb shrimp, peeled and deveined
- 2 cloves garlic, minced
- 1 tsp paprika
- ½ tsp chili flakes
- Juice of 1 lemon
- 2 tbsp olive oil
- ½ tsp salt
- ¼ tsp pepper
- 2 tbsp fresh parsley, finely chopped

Directions:

1. Create the zucchini noodles by using a spiral slicer to cut the zucchini into noodles and then place them into a colander over a bowl or in the sink
2. Sprinkle the zucchini with salt and toss to combine
3. Allow the zucchini to sit for 15 minutes while the salt extracts the excess moisture
4. In the meantime, combine the garlic, paprika, chili flakes, lemon juice and shrimp in a bowl, mix well
5. In a large skillet over medium high heat, add the olive oil
6. Once heated, add the shrimp and season with salt and pepper
7. Sauté until the shrimp is done, about 5 to 8 minutes
8. Rinse the zucchini under running water to remove the salt and dry on paper towels
9. Add the zucchini noodles and parsley to the garlic shrimp, toss to coat and serve
10. Enjoy!

Macros Per Serving – Calories:231 |Total Fat: 9.7g | Protein: 26.8g| **Net Carbs: 8.4g**

Salmon Stuffed Avocado

Your everyday avocado just got a delicious update! Stuffed with flaky salmon, this simple dish makes for an amazing lunch!

Prep Time: 10 Minutes
Cook Time: 20 Minutes
Total Time: 30 Minutes
Serves: 6

Ingredients:
- 2 small medium or 1 large avocado, seed removed
- 2 small salmon fillets - 6.2 oz cooked
- 1 small white onion, finely chopped
- ¼ cup sour cream or crème fraîche or mayonnaise
- 2 tbsp fresh lemon juice
- 1 tbsp ghee or coconut oil
- 1-2 tbsp dill, freshly chopped
- Salt, to taste
- Freshly ground black pepper, to taste

Garnish:
- Lemon wedges

Directions:
1. Preheat the oven to 400 degrees F
2. Place the salmon filets on a baking tray lined with parchment paper
3. Drizzle with melted ghee or olive oil, then season with salt and pepper and 1 tbsp of fresh lemon juice
4. Place in the oven and bake for 20 to 25 minutes
5. Once done, remove from the oven and allow it to cool down for 5-10 minutes
6. Using a fork, shred the salmon fillets and discard of the skin
7. In a bowl, add the shredded salmon with the finely chopped onion, sour cream and freshly chopped dill, a squeeze of lemon juice and season with salt and pepper to taste
8. Scoop out the middle of the avocado, leaving ½ to 1 inch of avocado
9. Cut the scooped-out avocado into smaller pieces and place it into the bowl with the salmon, mix well to combine
10. Fill each avocado half with the salmon and avocado mixture, add lemon
11. Enjoy!

Macros Per Serving – Calories: 463 | Total Fat: 34.6g | Protein: 27g | **Net Carbs: 6.4g**

Chipotle Steak Bowl

This beef stew is so rich in flavor and has everything you want - tender beef chucks and perfectly cooked vegetables!

Prep Time: 15 Minutes
Cook Time: 8 Minutes
Total Time: 23 Minutes
Serves 4

Ingredients:

- 16 oz. skirt steak
- Salt, to taste
- Pepper, to taste
- 4 oz. pepper jack cheese
- 1 cup sour cream
- 1 handful fresh cilantro
- 1 splash Chipotle Tabasco Sauce
- 1-2 cups of guacamole (homemade or store-brought)

Directions:

1. Prepare the skirt steak by seasoning it with a sprinkle of salt and pepper
2. Place a cast iron skillet on high heat, once it's hot, cook the skirt steak for 3-4 minutes on each side
3. Transfer the steak to rest on a plate for about 5 minutes
4. Slice the skirt steak against the grain into thin, bite-sized strips and divide into 4 portions, season to taste
5. Shred the pepper jack cheese using a cheese grater and top on each portion of skirt steak
6. Add about 1/4 cup of guacamole to each portion
7. Then add 1/4 cup of sour cream
8. Top with the optional Chipotle Tabasco Sauce and fresh cilantro
9. Enjoy!

Macros Per Serving – Calories:620 |Total Fat: 50g | Protein: 33g| **Net Carbs: 5.5g**

Grilled Lemon Herb Mediterranean Chicken Salad

Full of Mediterranean flavors - olives, tomatoes, cucumber, avocados, and chicken – this salad is a complete meal in a bowl!

Prep Time: 10 Minutes
Cook Time: 15 Minutes
Total Time: 25 Minutes
Serves: 4

Ingredients:
- 1 lbs skinless, boneless chicken thigh fillets (or chicken breasts)

For the marinade/ dressing:
- 2 tbsp olive oil
- Juice of 1 lemon or 1/4 cup fresh squeezed lemon juice
- 2 tbsp water
- 2 tbsp red wine vinegar
- 2 tbsp fresh chopped parsley
- 2 tsp dried basil
- 2 tsp garlic, minced
- 1 tsp dried oregano
- 1 tsp salt
- cracked pepper, to taste

For the salad:
- 4 cups Romaine or Cos lettuce leaves, washed and dried
- 1 large cucumber, diced
- 2 Roma tomatoes, diced
- 1 red onion, sliced
- 1 avocado, sliced
- 1/3 cup pitted Kalamata olives or black olives, sliced (optional)
- Lemon wedges to serve

Directions:
1. In a large jug, add whisk together the olive oil, lemon juice, water, red wine vinegar, chopped parsley, dried basil, garlic, oregano, salt and pepper
2. Pour half of the marinade into a large shallow dish, and then reserve the remaining dressing in a refrigerator for salad
3. Add the chicken to the marinade in the bowl, allow to marinade chicken for 15 to 30 minutes (or up to two hours in the refrigerator if time allows) - discard of the marinade once done

4. In the meantime, prepare the salad by mixing together the lettuce, tomatoes, red onions, avocado, and olives in a large salad bowl.
5. Once the chicken is ready, add 1 tbsp of oil in a grill pan or a grill plate over medium-high heat Grill chicken on both sides until browned and cooked through
6. Allow chicken to rest for 5 minutes, slice and arrange over salad
7. Drizzle salad with the remaining UNTOUCHED dressing in refridge
8. Serve with lemon wedges

Macros Per Serving – Calories:336 |Total Fat: 21g | Protein: 24g| **Net Carbs: 3g**

Blackened Steak Salad

A fresh salad with a hearty amount of steak and veggies sounds really good, right? What are you waiting for! Make it today!

Prep Time: 5 Minutes
Cook Time: 35 Minutes
Total Time: 40 Minutes
Serves: 4

Ingredients:
- 1 ½ lb flat iron steak, sliced into 1/2 -inch thick strips
- 2 tbsp butter
- 1 medium onion, thinly sliced
- 2 cloves garlic, minced
- 4 large mushrooms, thinly sliced
- 1 large head romaine lettuce, shredded
- 2 cups packed fresh spinach leaves
- 1 cup blue cheese crumbles
- 16 grape tomatoes, halved
- 1 medium orange bell pepper, sliced
- 1 medium yellow bell pepper, sliced
- 1 medium avocado, peeled, pitted, and sliced
- 4 tbsp olive oil
- 2 tsp smoked paprika
- 1 ½ tsp garlic powder
- 1 ½ tsp onion powder
- 1 ½ tsp dried thyme
- ½ tsp cayenne pepper
- ½ tsp dried basil
- ½ tsp ground cumin
- ½ tsp celery salt
- ¼ tsp dried oregano leaves
- Sea salt, to taste
- Black pepper, to taste

Directions:
1. In a large mixing bowl, toss the steak strips in 2 tbsp of olive oil
2. In a small mixing bowl, add the paprika, garlic powder, onion powder, thyme, cayenne pepper, basil, cumin, celery salt and oregano, mix to combine
3. Sprinkle the seasoning over the top of the steak in the bowl, toss until the meat is completely coated, set aside
4. In a large sauté pan over medium-low heat, add the remaining 2 tbsp of olive oil and the butter
5. Once heated, add the onion, garlic, and sea salt and black pepper to taste, sauté until the onion is a nice caramel color, about 20 minutes
6. Add in the mushrooms, sauté until they are soft and have released their liquid, about 10 minutes
7. In the meantime, divide the romaine and spinach among 4 plates
8. Top each plate of lettuce with one quarter of the blue cheese crumbles, tomatoes, orange and yellow bell pepper, and avocado
9. Line each of the topping in its own individual row
10. Heat the oven on broil, line the steak strips in a single layer on a broiling pan, broil on high for 5 minutes, or until the meat has reached the desired level of doneness
11. Then divide the cooked steak strips evenly among all 4 plates
12. Top with the caramelized onion and mushrooms
13. Enjoy!

Macros Per Serving – Calories:765 |Total Fat: 56g | Protein: 47g| **Net Carbs: 4g**

Tuna Cakes

These super simple Tuna Cakes are an easy meal you can quickly make in 15 minutes with just a few ingredients!

Prep Time: 5 Minutes
Cook Time: 10 Minutes
Total Time: 15 Minutes
Serves: 6

Ingredients:

2 (5 oz) cans of tuna packed in water
2 eggs
½ cup shredded cheese
4 oz pork rinds ground up into crumbs
2 tbsp Pico de Gallo, chopped onion, tomato and a little bit of jalapeño

Directions:

1. Open the cans of tuna, drain the liquid
2. Pulse the pork rinds in a food process until they become small crumbs
3. In a small bowl, combine the eggs, cheese, pork rinds, pico de gallo, and tuna, mix it fully combined
4. Divide the mixture into six equal parts, press the dough into small round patties
5. Fry the tuna cakes in coconut oil for a few minutes on each side, or until golden brown
6. Serve warm and enjoy!

Macros Per Serving – Calories:205 |Total Fat: 11.5g | Protein: 22.6g| **Net Carbs: 1g**

Hearty Chicken Soup

Comforting and healthy, this chicken soup is loaded with protein and low carb veggies that are so filling!

Prep Time: 10 Minutes
Cook Time: 35 Minutes
Total Time: 45 Minutes
Serves 8

Ingredients:
- 10 cups bone broth or chicken stock
- ½ tsp garlic powder
- ½ tsp dried oregano
- 1 cup thinly sliced celery
- ¼ cup chopped fresh parsley
- 1 tbsp apple cider vinegar
- 4 cups cooked, shredded or chopped chicken
- 1 ½ cups diced butternut squash
- 2 cups jicama, peeled and chopped small rice like pieces
- Sea salt, to taste
- Pepper, to taste

Directions:
1. In a large pot, combine the broth, garlic powder, dried oregano, celery, butternut squash and jicama
2. Bring to a boil, then lower heat and simmer uncovered for 30 minutes, or until veggies are fork tender
3. Add the chicken and cook for another 5 minutes, or until heated through - making sure not to overcook the chicken
4. Remove from the heat
5. Add the parsley and apple cider vinegar
6. Season with sea salt and pepper to taste
7. Serve!

Macros Per Serving – Calories:190 |Total Fat: 5g | Protein: 26g| **Net Carbs: 4g**

Egg Roll in a Bowl

All of the delicious flavors of your favorite fried Chinese appetizer in a bowl!

Prep Time: 15 Minutes
Cook Time: 10-15 Minutes
Total Time: 20-30 Minutes
Serves: 4

Ingredients:

For the "egg roll":
- 1 lb. ground chicken or pork sausage or ½ lb of each
- 2 cup coleslaw mix
- 1 cup sui choy or baby bok choy, shredded
- 1 cup bean sprouts

For the sauce:
- 1 tsp minced garlic
- 2 tbsp toasted sesame oil
- ½ – 1 tbsp fresh ginger, finely grated
- 1 tbsp rice vinegar (be sure it is sugar free!)
- 2 tbsp Braggs or coconut aminos or tamari or soy sauce

Directions:
1. Place a large high-sided skillet over medium-high heat, add the chicken or sausage meat and cook, crumbling the meat while it cooks, about 5 minutes
2. In the meantime, create the sauce by adding the minced garlic, sesame oil, fresh ginger, rice vinegar, coconut aminos or soy sauce to a small bowl whisk with a fork
3. Once the meat is cooked, remove from heat and drain some of the excess fat, leave about ¼ cup in the pan or enough to cook the rest of the dish without burning
4. Return skillet to heat, scrape up brown bits from the bottom of the pan with a wooden spatula. Reduce heat to medium, add in the coleslaw mix, asian vegetables and bean sprouts
5. Season with salt and black pepper, to taste, and cook, stirring frequently, until the vegetables wilt, about 4 to 5 minutes
6. Pour in the sauce mix, stir to combine for 1 minute or until heated through
7. Remove from heat, transfer to a serving platter or bowl
8. Garnish with chopped green onions and a sprinkle of sesame seeds

Macros Per Serving – Calories:322 |Total Fat: 23g | Protein: 17g| **Net Carbs: 8g**

Dinner

General Tso's Chicken

Way better than takeout, this recipe for general tso's chicken is made with a delicious homemade sauce! Just finish with fresh green onion and serve with cauliflower rice.

Prep Time: 15 Minutes
Cook Time: 15 Minutes
Total Time: 30 Minutes
Serves: 4

Ingredients:
- 2 lbs skinless boneless chicken thighs, chopped into 1 in pieces

For the marinade:
- 2 tbsp dry sherry
- 1 tbsp ginger, grated
- 3 cloves garlic
- ½ tsp salt
- ¼ tsp white pepper

For the chicken sauce:
- ¾ cup low sodium chicken broth
- 3 tbsp dry sherry
- 3 tbsp reduced sodium soy sauce
- 1 tbsp tomato paste
- 1 ½ tbsp rice wine vinegar

For the stir fry:
- 6 dried chili peppers
- 1 tsp toasted sesame oil
- 1 tsp sesame seeds
- 3 green onions

Directions:
1. In a bowl, prepare the marinade by mixing together the dry sherry, ginger, garlic, salt and white pepper, add the cut-up chicken thighs and marinate for 30 minutes
2. Once the chicken is done marinating, stir fry the chicken using a little oil over a medium high heat for 3-5 minutes, then remove it from the pan and set aside
3. Add the sauce ingredients - chicken broth, dry sherry, soy sauce, tomato paste, rice wine vinegar to the wok or cast-iron skillet, reduce over medium heat for about 10 minutes
4. Then add in the chilis during the last three minutes

5. Return the cooked chicken to the pan with the sauce, add the toasted sesame oil and green onions and cook for one minute or until warmed through
6. Serve hot with a sprinkle of toasted sesame seeds.

Macros Per Serving – Calories:322 |Total Fat: 10g | Protein: 46g| **Net Carbs: 3g**

Philly Cheesesteak Stuffed Peppers

Made with roast beef, onions, and tender mushrooms, these easy to make Philly cheesesteak stuffed peppers are 100% low carb and delicious!

Prep Time: 10 Minutes
Cook Time: 30 Minutes
Total Time: 40 Minutes
Serves 2

Ingredients:
- 3 bell peppers, cut in half lengthwise, ribs and seeds removed
- 2 tbsp butter or bacon fat, divided
- 1 medium to large yellow onion, julienned
- 8 oz. crimini mushrooms, sliced
- 2 lbs roast beef sandwich cuts into strips or 4 boxes (9 oz. each) beef steaks
- 4 cloves garlic, minced
- 1 tsp mineral salt
- ½ tsp cayenne pepper
- ¾ cup mozzarella, provolone, or pepper jack cheese, shredded, divided

Optional:
- ¼ tsp red pepper flakes

Directions:
1. Preheat the oven to 400 degrees F
2. Grease a 9- by 13-inch dish
3. Then place the pepper halves in the dish and pre-bake for about 10 to 15 minutes, until soft
4. In the meanwhile, place skillet over medium-high heat and melt 1 tablespoon butter
5. Once heated, add the onions and mushrooms and sauté, stirring often, until the onions are translucent
6. Add the remaining butter, roast beef, garlic, salt, cayenne pepper, and red pepper flakes to the skillet Sauté for an additional 10 to 15 minutes, or until the onions are caramelized and meat is heated
7. Remove the peppers from the oven, add about 1 tbsp of cheese to the bottom of each pepper half
8. Stuff the peppers with the meat mixture, top with the remaining cheese
9. Bake for 10 to 15 minutes, or until cheese is melted and they begin to lightly brown
10. Enjoy!

Macros Per Serving – Calories:302 |Total Fat: 13g | Protein: 37g| **Net Carbs: 5g**

Cauliflower Rice with King Crab

Made with Asian inspired cauliflower rice and tender bits of king crab, this yummy fried rice recipe will soon be your favorite dinner dish!

Prep Time: 10 Minutes
Cook Time: 20 Minutes
Total Time: 30 Minutes
Serves 4

Ingredients:
- 1 lb (2 frozen) King crab legs
- 24 oz. riced cauliflower
- 1 tbsp sesame oil
- 2 large eggs, beaten
- pinch of salt
- ½ small onion, finely diced
- 2 garlic cloves, minced
- 5 scallions, diced, whites and greens separated
- 3 tbsp coconut aminos
- Cooking spray

Directions:
1. Prepare the cauliflower rice by placing a few florets at a time into the food processor and pulse until the cauliflower is small and resembles the texture of rice or couscous – make sure you don't over process or it will be mushy, set aside the cauliflower rice and repeat with the remaining cauliflower florets in batches
2. In a large pot, add about 2 inches of water and bring to a boil
3. Add in the crab leg and cook, covered until heated through for about 10 minutes
4. Once cooked, remove the crab from the shell and lightly flake, set aside
5. Add the egg to a bowl and seasoning with a pinch of salt, set aside
6. In a large skillet or wok over medium heat, spray with oil
7. Once heated, add the eggs and cook, turning a few times until set, then set aside
8. Reduce the heat to medium-low, add in the sesame oil and sauté the onions, scallion whites, and garlic for about 3 to 4 minutes, or until soft
9. Raise the heat to medium-high
10. Add in the cauliflower "rice" to the sauté pan with coconut aminos
11. Mix well, then cover and cook for approximately 5 to 6 minutes, stirring occasionally, until the cauliflower is slightly crispy on the outside and tender on the inside
12. Add the egg and crab, remove from heat and mix in scallion greens
13. Serve!

Macros Per Serving (1 ½ cups)– Calories:237 |Total Fat: 8g | Protein: 29.5g| **Net Carbs: 8g**

Chicken Tetrazzini

Craving pasta tonight? Make this amazing low carb chicken tetrazzini instead! It's made with zucchini noodles, a cream sauce, mushrooms and chicken breasts

Prep Time: 40 Minutes
Cook Time: 1 Hour
Total Time: 1 Hour 40 Minutes
Serves 2

Ingredients:
- 3 zucchinis, medium
- 2 tbsp butter
- ½ onion, diced
- 2 cups mushrooms, sliced
- 1 clove garlic, minced
- 2 chicken breasts boneless, skinless, chopped
- 1.5 cups heavy cream
- 1 tsp xantham gum
- ¼ cup mozzarella cheese shredded
- Salt, to sweat zucchini noodles
- Salt, to taste

Directions:
1. Prepare the noodles by spiralizing each zucchini into spaghetti noodle shapes using a spiralizer tool. Then add salt to the zucchini noodles and layout them over a folded paper towels to remove excess moisture. Allow the zucchini noodles to sit for 30 minutes, then squeeze them to remove any additional water
2. Preheat oven to 400 degrees F
3. In a large saucepan over medium heat, melt the butter
4. Once heated, add the onion, mushrooms, and garlic to the pan, stirring as needed
5. Once the onions become translucent, add the chopped chicken breast and increase temperature to medium-high
6. When the chicken cooks to white in color, add in the heavy cream and thoroughly mix, all while bringing the sauce to a boil
7. Once the cream is broiling, reduce the heat and allow the sauce to simmer for an additional 1 to 2 minutes
8. Remove the sauce from heat and whisk in the xantham gum little by little to thicken up - If you prefer a thinner, runnier sauce, leave it out or cut the amount in half
9. Arrange zucchini noodles in the bottom of a deep casserole dish, cover the entire bottom of the bakeware about an inch thick. Use a 9 x 6-inch dish for 10 servings of this recipe

10. Add the creamy chicken mushroom sauce on top of the zucchini noodles, smooth the mixture evenly over the top and distribute it throughout the casserole dish
11. Sprinkle mozzarella cheese on top
12. Bake for 40 minutes, until the top is brown
13. Enjoy

Recipe Notes – If you want to add more protein to this dish, add extra chicken breast to the recipe.

Macros Per Serving – Calories:194 |Total Fat: 16g | Protein: 7g| **Net Carbs: 4g**

Salmon Patties

Flavorful and moist, these Salmon Patties are super easy to make! Plus, you'll be enjoying them in no time!

Prep Time: 10 Minutes
Cook Time: 10 Minutes
Total Time: 20 Minutes
Serves: 6

Ingredients:
- 18 oz wild pink salmon, skinless and boneless (about 3 cans), well drained (see notes)
- 2 eggs
- ½ cup almond meal
- ½ cup fresh parsley, chopped
- 1 shallot, finely chopped
- 1 green onion, sliced
- 1 tsp salt
- 1 tsp garlic powder
- ½ tsp dill
- ¼ tsp black pepper
- 2 tbsp lime juice
- 2 tbsp olive oil

Directions:
1. In a medium bowl, flake the salmon apart, add the almond meal, parsley, shallot, green onion, salt, garlic powder, dill, black pepper, lime juice, and the eggs, mix well to combine
2. Form into 6 patties, use a ½ cup measuring cup making sure all the patties are the same size
3. Place a nonstick skillet over medium heat, add the olive oil
4. Fry the patties for 4 to 5 minutes on each side until golden brown and crispy
5. Serve with cilantro lime cauliflower rice

Recipe Notes – You can use fresh salmon too.
Macros Per Serving – Calories:232 |Total Fat: 14g | Protein: 22g| **Net Carbs: 2g**

Jamaican Curry Chicken

Full of Caribbean flavors, this low carb Jamaican Curry Chicken is perfect for dinner! Don't forget to serve it up with some cauliflower rice!

Total Time: 40 Minutes

Serves: 6

Ingredients:
- 2 lbs of chicken legs, cleaned
- 1 tsp seasoning salt
- 2 tbsp Jamaican curry powder
- 1 stalk of scallion
- ½ medium sized white onion
- 1 sprig of thyme

Directions:
1. Season the chicken thoroughly with the seasoning salt, add the curry powder, scallion, onion, and thyme
2. Spray a pan with nonstick to coat the skillet, place over high heat
3. Once hot, brown the chicken in the skillet for 10 minutes
4. Add 2 cups of water, cover and simmer for 30 minutes, stirring frequently

Macros Per Serving – Calories:198 |Total Fat: 6.8g | Protein: 30g| **Net Carbs: 2g**

Creamy Asparagus and Shrimp Alfredo

A decadent meal of shrimp and asparagus swimming in a delicious creamy Alfredo sauce, all while being low in carbs!

Prep Time: 1 Minute
Cook Time: 5 Minutes
Total Time: 7 Minutes
Serves: 4

Ingredients:
- 1 lb raw wild caught shrimp, peeled & deveined
- 2 tbsp organic grass-fed butter or ghee
- 1/3 cup grated parmesan cheese
- 2 cups fresh or frozen Asparagu
- 1 cup heavy cream
- Sea salt, to taste
- Black pepper, to tast

Directions:
1. Toss the shrimp with salt and pepper
2. In a skillet over medium heat, sauté shrimp in butter until opaque, about 2 to 3 minutes
3. Add asparagus, sauté 1 to 2 minutes
4. Add in the cream and cheese, reduce heat and stir until cheese is melted and sauce is thickened.
5. Serve immediately!

Macros Per Serving – Calories:412 |Total Fat: 33g | Protein: 26g| **Net Carbs: 0g**

Shredded Chicken Chili

Busy day? Enjoy this Shredded Chicken Chili when you're in need of a filling keto-friendly meal in a hurry!

Prep Time: 5 Minutes
Cook Time: 25 Minutes
Total Time: 30 Minutes
Serves 4

Ingredients:
- 4 chicken breasts large, shredded
- 1 tbsp butter
- ½ onion chopped
- 2 cups chicken broth
- 10 oz. diced tomatoes canned, undrained
- 2 oz. tomato paste
- 1 tbsp chili powder
- 1 tbsp cumin
- ½ tbsp garlic powder
- 4 oz. cream cheese
- Salt, to taste
- Pepper to taste

Optional:
- 1 jalapeño pepper, chopped
- Monterey jack cheese, toppings
- Cilantro, toppings

Directions:
1. Prepare the chicken by boiling chicken breasts in water or broth on stovetop that covers the breasts for 10 to 12 minutes. Once the meat is no longer pink, remove from the pot and shred with two forks
2. In a large stockpot over medium-high heat, melt the butter
3. Once heated, add the onion and cook until translucent
4. Add in the shredded chicken, chicken broth, diced tomatoes, tomato paste, chili powder, cumin, garlic powder, and jalapeño to the pot, stir gently to combine
5. Bring to a boil, then turn the heat down to a simmer over medium-low heat and cover for 10 minutes
6. Cut the cream cheese into small, 1-inch chunks
7. Remove the lid and mix in the cream cheese, increase the heat back up to medium-high and continue to stir until the cream cheese is completely blended in
8. Remove chili from heat and season with salt and pepper to taste
9. Enjoy!

Macros Per Serving – Calories:201 |Total Fat: 11g | Protein: 18g| **Net Carbs: 6g**

Garlic Butter Brazilian Steak

This recipe for Garlic Butter Brazilian Steak makes the juiciest and most tender steaks with a golden garlic butter sauce. Plus, it only takes 15 minutes!

Prep Time: 10 Minute
Cook Time: 5 Minutes
Total Time: 15 Minutes
Serves: 4

Ingredients:
- 1 ½ lbs skirt steak trimmed and cut into 4 pieces
- Freshly ground black pepper
- 2 tbsp canola oil or vegetable oil
- 2 oz unsalted butter, 4 tbsp
- 1 tbs chopped fresh flat-leaf parsley
- 6 medium cloves garlic
- Kosher salt

Directions:
1. Peel the garlic cloves, smash them with the side of a chef's knife and sprinkle the garlic lightly with salt and mince it
2. Pat the steak dry, season generously on both sides with salt and pepper
3. Place a heavy-duty 12-inch skillet, add the oil
4. Once heated, add the steak and brown well on both sides, 2 to 3 minutes per side for medium rare
5. Transfer the steak to a plate and allow to rest while you make the garlic butter
6. In an 8-inch skillet, melt the butter over low heat, add the garlic and cook, swirling the pan frequently, until lightly golden, about 4 minutes
7. Lightly salt to taste
8. Slice the steak, if desired, and transfer to 4 plates
9. Spoon the garlic butter over the steak, sprinkle with the parsley, and serve

Macros Per Serving – Calories:428 |Total Fat: 31g | Protein: 37g| **Net Carbs: 1g**

Pork Chops Smothered in Caramelized Onion & Bacon

In under an hour you can enjoy a juicy, tender pork chops smothered in a creamy onion and bacon sauce!

Prep Time: 10 Minutes
Cook Time: 45 Minutes
Total Time: 55 Minutes
Serves 4

Ingredients:
- 6 slices bacon chopped
- 2 small onions thinly sliced
- ¼ tsp salt
- ¼ pepper
- 4 bone-in pork chops 1 inch thick
- Salt, to taste
- Pepper to taste
- ½ cup chicken broth
- ¼ cup heavy cream

Directions:
1. In a large sauté pan over medium heat, cook bacon until crispy
2. Once cooked, use a slotted spoon to transfer to a bowl, reserve the bacon grease
3. Add the onions to bacon grease, season with salt and pepper, cook, stirring frequently for 10 minutes, until onions are soft and golden brown, then place the onions in the bowl with the bacon
4. Increase the heat to medium high and season the pork chops with salt and pepper
5. Add the chops to pan and brown on one side for 3 minutes, then turn the chops over and reduce the heat to medium, cooking on the other side until internal temperature reaches 135 degrees F, for about 7 to 10 more minutes
6. Transfer the pork chops to a plate and tent with foil
7. Add the broth to pan and scrape up the browned bits
8. Add the cream and simmer until mixture is thickened, for about 2 to 3 minutes Return the onions and bacon back to the pan, stir to combine
9. Top the pork chops with onion and bacon sauce
10. Serve!

Macros Per Serving – Calories:342 |Total Fat: 18g | Protein: 37g| **Net Carbs: 5.28g**

Creamy Garlic Chicken Soup

Garlicy and creamy, this comforting soup is so easy to make on a chilly night.

Prep Time: 10 Minutes
Cook Time: 10 Minutes
Total Time: 20 Minutes
Serves 2

Ingredients:
- 2 tbsp butter
- 2 cups shredded chicken, about 1 large chicken breast
- 4 oz. cream cheese cubed
- 2 tbsp garlic seasoning
- 14.5 oz. chicken broth
- ¼ cup heavy cream
- Salt, to taste

Directions:
1. In a saucepan over medium heat, melt butter
2. Once heated, add in the shredded chicken to pan and coat with melted butter
3. As chicken heats up, add in the cubes of cream cheese and garlic gusto seasoning. mix well to combine
4. Once the cream cheese is melted and evenly distributed, add in the chicken broth and heavy cream
5. Bring to a boil, then reduce heat to low and simmer for 3 to 4 minutes
6. Season with the salt to taste
7. Serve!

Recipe Notes – Create the garlic gusto seasoning by combing a mix of parsley, garlic, onion, lemon peel and paprika.

Macros Per Serving – Calories:307 |Total Fat: 25g | Protein: 33g| **Net Carbs: 4g**

Roasted Lemon Chicken

Covered in an herb butter sauce, this roasted lemon chicken recipe is easy to make and pairs well with your favorite veggies.

Prep Time: 5 Minutes
Cook Time: 35 Minutes
Total Time: 40 Minutes
Serves 4

Ingredients:
- 1 ¼ lb boneless skinless chicken breasts
- 1 tbsp olive oil
- 1 tsp Italian seasoning
- 3 tbsp butter, melted
- 1 tsp minced garlic
- ¼ cup chicken broth
- 2 tbsp lemon juice
- 1 tbsp chopped parsley
- Salt, to taste
- Pepper, to taste

Optional:
- Lemon slices, for serving

Directions:
1. Preheat the oven to 400 degrees F
2. Season the chicken breasts on both sides with salt, pepper and the Italian seasoning
3. In a large pan over medium high heat, add the olive oil
4. Once heated, add the chicken breasts and cook for 3 to 5 minutes on each side or until browned, then transfer the chicken to a baking dish
5. In a small bowl, mix together the butter, garlic, chicken broth and lemon juice, pour the butter mixture over the chicken
6. Bake for 25 minutes or until chicken is cooked through, true bake time will depend on the thickness of the chicken breasts
7. Spoon the sauce on the bottom of the baking dish over the chicken, then sprinkle with parsley
8. Serve and garnish with lemon slices

Recipe Notes – If your chicken breasts are less than 1 inch thick, then decrease the bake time accordingly.

Macros Per Serving – Calories: 271 | Total Fat: 15g | Protein: 30g | **Net Carbs: 0g**

Cheesy Zucchini Gratin Casserole

Creamy and really cheesy, this super easy Zucchini Gratin Casserole will be an instant hit! Plus, it's made with just 6 main ingredients.

Prep Time: 10 Minutes
Cook Time: 45 Minutes
Total Time: 55 Minutes
Serves 9

Ingredients:
- 4 cups sliced raw zucchini
- 1 small onion, peeled and sliced thin
- 1 ½ cups shredded pepper jack cheese
- 2 tbsp butter
- ½ tsp garlic powder
- ½ cup heavy whipping cream
- Salt, to taste
- Pepper, to taste

Directions:
1. Preheat oven to 375 degrees F
2. Grease a 9×9 or equivalent oven proof pan
3. Overlap 1/3 of the zucchini and onion slices in the greased pan, season with salt and pepper and then sprinkle with 1/2 cup of shredded cheese
4. Repeat two more times until there are at least three layers and you have used up all of the zucchini, onions, and shredded cheese
5. In a microwave safe bowl, combine the garlic powder, butter, and heavy cream
6. Heat for one minute or until the butter has melted, stir to mix
7. Gently pour the butter and cream mixture over the zucchini layers
8. Bake for about 45 minutes, or until the liquid has thickened and the top is golden brown
9. Serve!

Recipe Notes – Depending on your zucchini, you may have to cook it longer in order to reduce the sauce. If you find that it is very watery after the 45 minutes, lower the oven temp to 350 degrees F and cook for another 10 minutes or so.

Macros Per Serving – Calories:230 |Total Fat: 20g | Protein: 8g| **Net Carbs: 3g**

Classic Italian Meatballs

Make classic Italian meatballs a low-carb dinner with this juicy and tender meatball recipe!!

Prep Time: 15 Minutes
Cook Time: 20 Minutes
Total Time: 35 Minutes
Serves 4-5

Ingredients:
- ½ lb ground beef chuck, 85 % lean
- ½ lb ground pork, turkey or veal
- ¼ cup Parmesan cheese, grated
- ¼ cup heavy cream
- 1 large egg, beaten
- 2 tbsp fresh parsley, minced
- 1 tbsp onion, finely grated
- 1 clove garlic, grated
- ½ tsp salt
- ¼ tsp pepper

Optional Sauce:
- 2 cups your favorite low carb marinara sauce

Directions:
1. In a medium bowl, add the beef and pork, and break up into smaller chunks, aiming to create an even mix
2. Add parmesan cheese, heavy cream, beaten egg, parsley, finely grated onion, garlic, salt and pepper to the meat and mix with a hand mixer until combined - don't over-mix
3. Lightly oil your hands and roll the meat into 12 meatballs, set aside
4. Place a large frying pan over medium heat, add 1-2 tsp of oil and swirl it to coat the pan
5. Once hot, add the meatballs to the pan, making sure they don't touch or overcrowd it
6. Cook the meatballs for approximately 1 1/2 minutes per side, turning at least 4 times
7. Cook for 10 to 15 minutes, until brown and then transfer the meatballs to a plate
8. Heat the sauce in the same pan, scraping up the brown bits for a flavorful sauce or warm the sauce on the stove and pour over the meatballs
9. Garnish with parsley
10. Serve with zoodles or top with mozzarella cheese and melt it under the broiler

Macros Per Serving – Calories:387 |Total Fat: 22g | Protein: 19g| **Net Carbs: 1g**

Italian Sausage with Peppers and Onions in Marinara Sauce

Sweet Italian sausage, colorful bell peppers and onions covered in a marinara sauce, oh it so good alone or served with a keto-friendly side!

Prep Time: 10 Minutes
Cook Time: 20 Minutes
Total Time: 30 Minutes
Serves 4

Ingredients:
- 1 lb Italian sausage links
- 9 oz mixed color bell pepper, sliced into strips (about 2 large peppers)
- 2 oz sliced onion (about ½ cup)
- 1 tbsp olive oil (or more to taste)
- 1 tsp minced garlic
- ½ cup Rao's Marinara Sauce
- Salt, to taste
- Pepper, to taste

Directions:
1. In a large skillet over medium heat, add the 1 1/2 tsp oil
2. Once heated, add the sausage slices and brown for about 8-10 minutes
3. Transfer the sausage to a plate
4. In a clean pan, heat the 1 tsp of oil over medium heat
5. Once hot, sauté the bell peppers and onion with the minced garlic until softened about 10 minutes
6. Add the sausage and any juices back to the pan to re-heat
7. Add the Marinara sauce, stir to coat
8. Taste and season with salt and pepper
9. Serve!

Macros Per Serving – Calories:420 |Total Fat: 32.5g | Protein: 23.5g| **Net Carbs: 6.5g**

Easy Shrimp Scampi

Just add the ingredients to a foil packet and you'll have a delicious Shrimp Scampi meal in 20 minutes!

Prep Time: 10 Minutes
Cook Time: 10 Minutes
Total Time: 20 Minutes
Serves 4

Ingredients:
- 40 jumbo shrimp, peeled and deveined, about 1 lb
- 2 tbsp unsalted butter, melted
- 4 garlic cloves, 2 grated, 2 thinly sliced
- ½ tsp kosher salt
- 1 tbsp extra virgin olive oil
- ¼ cup dry white wine
- 1 tbsp fresh lemon juice
- 4 pinches red pepper flakes
- 3 tbsp chopped parsley
- 1 lemon, cut into wedges

Other:
- Heavy-duty aluminum foil

Directions:
1. In a medium bowl, whisk together the grated garlic, salt and oil
2. Add in the shrimp, toss to coat, and chill, uncovered for at least 30 minutes or for 1 hour
3. Make the foil packets by tearing off 4 16" sheets of aluminum foil
4. Place 10 shrimp on the center of each foil sheet, then top each with the remaining garlic slices, 1 tbsp wine, lemon juice, a pinch of red pepper flakes and 1/2 tbsp melted butter over each
5. Close the packets by bringing up the long sides of the foil, so the ends meet over the food, then double fold the ends, leaving enough room for heat to circulate inside. Then double fold the two short ends to seal the packet
6. Grill over high heat, 8 minutes, using gloves or tongs to remove and carefully open it or bake the packets in the oven, preheat the oven to 425 degrees F for 10 minutes
7. Top the shrimp with chopped parsley
8. Serve with lemon wedges
9. Serve with your favorite keto-friendly side

Macros Per Serving – Calories:224 |Total Fat: 11g | Protein: 24g| **Net Carbs: 4.5g**

Beef Stuffed Zucchini Boats

In the mood for a little Italian? Try this recipe for Beef Stuffed Zucchini Boats made with a flavorful marinara and cheese served on top of zucchini.

Prep Time: 15 Minutes
Cook Time: 20 Minutes
Total Time: 35 Minutes
Serves: 6

Ingredients:
- 6-8 medium zucchini or 12 small
- 1 lb ground beef
- 1 tbsp olive oil
- ½ cup onion chopped
- 2 cloves garlic minced
- 1 cup marinara sauce
- 1 tbsp Italian seasoning
- ¼ tsp salt
- ¼ tsp pepper
- 1 cup low-fat shredded cheddar or mozzarella cheese

Directions:
1. Preheat oven to 375 degrees F
2. Slice the zucchini in half, and carve them out with a spoon, set pulp aside
3. Chop the zucchini, and set it aside
4. Line the zucchini boats on a baking sheet lined with parchment paper or lightly greased with oil
5. Place a non-skillet over medium heat, add the olive oil
6. Once heated, add the onion, cook onion for 2 to 3 minutes or until it begins to golden
7. Then add the garlic, cook for a few seconds
8. Add the ground beef, cook until it's no longer pink, 3 to 5 minutes
9. Then dd the marinara sauce, zucchini pulp, Italian seasoning, salt and pepper, simmer for 8 to 10 minutes
10. Spoon mixture into zucchini boats and top each with a drizzle of cheese
11. Bake for 15 to 20 minutes or until the cheese is fully melted and bubbly
12. Enjoy!

Macros Per Serving – Calories:330 |Total Fat: 22g | Protein: 7g| **Net Carbs: 1g**

Rainbow Vegetable Noodles

Why not dig into a beautiful plate of colorful roasted rainbow vegetable noodles for dinner!

Prep Time: 15 Minutes
Cook Time: 20 Minutes
Total Time: 35 Minutes
Serves 6

Ingredients:
- 1 medium zucchini
- 1 medium summer squash
- 1 large carrot
- 1 small sweet potato
- 4 oz red onion
- 6 oz mixed bell peppers
- 3 large cloves garlic
- 4 tbsp bacon fat, or olive oil, butter or ghee
- Sea salt, to taste
- Black pepper, to taste

Directions:
1. Preheat oven to 400 degrees F
2. Coat a baking sheet with the bacon fat or olive oil, butter, or ghee
3. Using a spiral slicer, spiral the zucchini, squash, carrot and sweet potato into noodle-like ribbons.
4. Then use a mandolin, on the thinnest setting or a knife to slice the red onion, bell peppers, and garlic
5. In a bowl, add the vegetables, sprinkle with salt and pepper, and toss to combine
6. Spread the vegetable noodles in a thin layer across baking sheet
7. Bake for 20 minutes, tossing after 10 minutes
8. Serve as a side

Macros Per Serving – Calories:128 |Total Fat: 9g | Protein: 2g| **Net Carbs: 8g**

Zucchini Noodles with Garlic Shrimp

Toss together Zucchini noodles and delicious garlic shrimp, and enjoy a healthy meal in 20 minutes!

Prep Time: 15 Minutes
Cook Time: 6 Minutes
Total Time: 21 Minutes
Serves 4

Ingredients:
- 6 zucchini, washed
- 1 lb shrimp, peeled and deveined
- 2 cloves garlic, minced
- 1 tsp paprika
- ½ tsp chili flakes
- Juice of 1 lemon
- 2 tbsp olive oil
- ½ tsp salt
- ¼ tsp pepper
- 2 tbsp fresh parsley, finely chopped

Directions:
1. Create the zucchini noodles by using a spiral slicer to cut the zucchini into noodles and then place them into a colander over a bowl or in the sink
2. Sprinkle the zucchini with salt and toss to combine
3. Allow the zucchini to sit for 15 minutes while the salt extracts the excess moisture
4. In the meantime, combine the garlic, paprika, chili flakes, lemon juice and shrimp in a bowl, mix well
5. In a large skillet over medium high heat, add the olive oil
6. Once heated, add the shrimp and season with salt and pepper
7. Sauté until the shrimp is done, about 5 to 8 minutes
8. Rinse the zucchini under running water to remove the salt and dry on paper towels
9. Add the zucchini noodles and parsley to the garlic shrimp, toss to coat and serve
10. Enjoy!

Macros Per Serving – Calories:231 |Total Fat: 9.7g | Protein: 26.8g| **Net Carbs: 8.4g**

Maple Walnut Crusted Salmon

Topped with a sweet syrup pecan crust, this flaky salmon is great for dinner!

Prep Time: 5 Minutes 2-3 Hours
Cook Time: 10 Minutes
Total Time: 15 Minutes, 2-3 Hours
Serves 4

Ingredients:
- 2 tbsp ghee, for pan
- 6 oz. salmon fillets
- A pinch of salt
- A pinch of pepper

Maple Walnut Crust:
- ½ cup finely chopped walnuts
- 1 tsp smoked paprika
- ½ tsp chipotle powder
- ½ tsp onion powder
- ½ tsp cracked black pepper
- 3 tbsp Sukrin gold fiber syrup or alternative syrup
- 1 tbsp apple cider vinegar
- 1 tsp coconut aminos

Directions:
1. Prepare the maple walnut crust by combining the finely chopped walnuts, smoked paprika, chipotle powder, onion powder, black pepper, Sukrin gold fiber syrup, apple cider vinegar and coconut aminos in a small bowl, stir well to combine
2. Place the salmon fillets on a plate and spoon the walnut mixture over each piece of fish, distributing it evenly
3. Place in the refrigerator, uncovered, for 2 to 3 hours.
4. Preheat the oven to 425 degrees F
5. In a large oven-safe skillet over high heat, add the ghee
6. Once heated, add the pieces of fish and allow them to cook undisturbed for about 2 minutes, allowing the skin to sear
7. Transfer the salmon from the pan to the oven and continue cooking the fish for about 5-8 minutes, depending on desired doneness and thickness of the fillets
8. Drizzle the salmon with some of the melted ghee and additional syrup for serving, if desired

Macros Per Serving – Calories:443 |Total Fat: 27.3g | Protein: 40.2g| **Net Carbs: 10.9g**

Conclusion & FAQ

Now, we've come to the end of my cookbook! So far, you've learned how the keto diet works and have plenty of recipes to cook on your journey into ketosis. If you have any questions, check out my helpful FAQ section that will give you all the important answers!

Q: How Long Until I Get into Ketosis?
A: It will take time for your body to go into a ketosis state. But if you really stick to your new keto diet, you can get into ketosis in around 2-7 days depending on what you're eating, your body type and overall activity level.
Helpful tip! You can actually get into ketosis faster by exercising on an empty stomach, and if you restrict your carb intake to just 20g or less a day, and by keeping a note of your water intake.

Q. How Do I Track My Carb Intake?
A. Download a helpful carb counting mobile app to track them anywhere. Or you can find out your net carbs by subtracting your total fiber intake from your carb intake.
Do I Have to Count All of My Calories?
You don't really have to worry about calories on the keto diet because the fats and proteins you'll be consuming will keep you fuller longer.
Now, if you're exercising regularly (like you should), be aware that exercising can create a larger calorie deficit than what it's supposed to be. If this happens, then you'll have to make it up with food. Other than that, please stick to eating properly, and be sure not to go too far into a food deficit.

Q: Can I Really Eat Too Much Fat?
A: Yes, you can overindulge and eat too much fat. Eating too much fat will push you over your calorie deficit and turn into a calorie surplus. Most people don't over eat on a high fat low-carb diet, but it can happen.

Q: How Much Weight Will I Lose?
A: How much weight you lose depends on you. If you're exercising, cutting out foods that slow your results like artificial sweeteners, wheat products, and dairy, it will help. Water weight loss is also common and it shows that your body is just starting to become a fat burning machine.

Q: I Just Started and I Don't Feel So Good. What Can I Do?
A: It's common for keto beginners to get headaches and "brain fogginess". This is because ketosis works like a diuretic and you'll lose electrolytes that you really need to replace. As

you transition from your regular diet into ketosis, stay hydrated and consume salt by making a broth, or eating salty foods like bacon, salted nuts, or deli cold cuts.

Q: How Do I Know If I'm in Ketosis or Not?

A: The best way to know if you're in ketosis or not is with a blood ketone meter. Another way is with test strips that will give you a general idea of your ketosis state (these also tend to be pretty inaccurate).

- **Light Ketosis**: 0.5 mmol/L – 0.8 mmol/L
- **Medium Ketosis**: 0.9 mmol/L – 1.4 mmol/L
- **Deep Ketosis** (this one is best for weight loss): 1.5 mmol/L – 3.0 mmol/L

Q: Can I Drink Alcohol?

A: You can enjoy alcohol, but you have to be careful. Wine, beer, and cocktails all have carbohydrates. As a rule of thumb, stick to clear liquors as they have fewer carbs.

Printed in Great Britain
by Amazon